The Use and Misuse of Psychiatric Drugs

The Use and Misuse of Psychiatric Drugs
An Evidence-Based Critique

Joel Paris
MD
Professor of Psychiatry
McGill University
Montreal
Canada

WILEY-BLACKWELL

A John Wiley & Sons, Ltd, Publication

This edition first published 2010, © 2010 John Wiley & Sons, Ltd.

Wiley-Blackwell is an imprint of John Wiley & Sons, Ltd, formed by the merger of Wiley's global Scientific, Technical and Medical business with Blackwell Publishing.

Registered office: John Wiley & Sons, Ltd, The Atrium, Southern Gate, Chichester, West Sussex, PO19 8SQ, UK

Other Editorial Offices:
9600 Garsington Road, Oxford, OX4 2DQ, UK
111 River Street, Hoboken, NJ 07030-5774, USA

For details of our global editorial offices, for customer services and for information about how to apply for permission to reuse the copyright material in this book please see our website at www.wiley.com/wiley-blackwell

Library of Congress Cataloging-in-Publication Data

Paris, Joel, 1940-
   The use and misuse of psychiatric drugs : an evidence-based critique / Joel Paris.
      p. ; cm.
   Includes index.
   ISBN 978-0-470-74571-7 (pbk.)
  1. Psychopharmacology.   2. Psychotropic drugs.   3. Evidence-based psychiatry.   I. Title.
   [DNLM: 1. Psychotropic Drugs.   2. Evidence-Based Practice.   3. Psychopharmacology–standards.
4. Psychopharmacology.   QV 77.2 P232u 2010]
   RM315.P367 2010
   615′.78–dc22

                                                                                  2010018058

ISBN: 9780470745717 (P/B)

A catalogue record for this book is available from the British Library.

Set in 10.5/12.5 Times by Aptara Inc., New Delhi, India.
Printed in Singapore by Fabulous Printers Pte Ltd.

First Impression 2010

This book is dedicated to the students I have taught
(and who have taught me) over the last four decades

Contents

Foreword

Forty years ago, whenever new drugs were introduced into medicine they created great excitement and were all the rage. Now, each new agent also creates great excitement but instead just calls the rage. This is especially true of drugs for mental disorders. The rage is directed at those who create new diagnostic groupings that just medicalise normal distress, researchers who distort their findings for every reason apart from wanting to disseminate good science, pharmaceutical companies for doing anything and everything to extend their sales, and doctors for being so gullible to believe the nonsense that is peddled to them by all these other agencies. Are all these claims true and, if they are, who can we believe? Well, you could make a start by reading this book. Dr Paris is not a psychopharmacologist, a creator of diagnoses, an employee of a drug company, or a simple prescriber. He is a sophisticated psychiatrist with many years of experience and an excellent knowledge base. This book represents a well balanced, sober account of a serious issue that affects almost all of us in one way or another. His language is carefully chosen, his research is impeccable and his conclusions based on evidence. We can all learn from sorry chapters in the history of medicine and unless we take corrective action it will not be long before they fill book after book. Patients, health professionals, service planners and drug companies could all gain from the lessons of this text, so please read on – and prepare to be surprised.

Peter Tyrer
Head of Centre for Mental Health,
Imperial College, London W6 8RP

Introduction

WHAT THIS BOOK IS ABOUT

Many books have been written about the use of drugs in psychiatry. Large specialized research texts have probed deeply into the latest scientific data. Smaller books, some of which fit into the pocket of a lab coat, have offered practical hints for daily practice. Most volumes proclaim received wisdoms, celebrating the modern age of neuroscience and chemical therapy. Yet quite a few books have been broadsides *against* drug therapy, based on the idea that psychopharmacology is either a scam, or a conspiracy against social deviance.

This book is different. It will neither celebrate nor attack psychopharmacology. Nor is it designed to be a clinical guide to practice. Instead, it focuses on the *use* and *misuse* of psychiatric drugs. Its thesis is that pharmacological agents are highly effective when used properly, but can do harm when given without sufficient evidence to patients who will not benefit from them. It will argue that while most drugs in psychiatry are valuable, they are being over-prescribed. It will also suggest that most patients do not need to be treated with multiple drugs. In summary, this book will be respectful to good practice, and critical of bad or unproven interventions.

One factor behind the misuse of drugs is that the science behind psychopharmacology has been over-sold. I am as impressed as anyone else by the advances in neuroscience in recent decades. As a student, I was fascinated with this area of research, which was one of the reasons I went into psychiatry. However, neuroscience has not yet explained very much about mental illness. And in spite of the many interesting theories about the relation of drugs to neurotransmitters, we only have a general idea of how the agents we prescribe actually work.

The practice of psychopharmacology has outrun scientific data, and this book will criticize the "hype" that has come to afflict clinical work. The effectiveness of many drugs has been exaggerated through selective publication of clinical trials. The resulting excess of enthusiasm supports a serious over-prescription of drugs–both to adults and to children.

These problems relate to another theme of this book: how academic psychiatry (and academic medicine as a whole) has been corrupted by the pharmaceutical industry. In recent years, this issue has come to wide attention, both in the medical literature and the media. Senators and parliamentarians have raised public concern about how drugs are being developed and prescribed. While one can now read about these problems in the morning newspaper, there is little reason to believe that they are on the way to being solved.

To assess scientific support for the efficacy of psychiatric drugs, I have had to review an enormous literature. Many thousands of research papers have been published in the last 50 years. Yet only a minority of these studies meet the high standards of modern evidence-based medicine. I have therefore focused on data drawn from randomized controlled trials, sophisticated effectiveness studies, and meta-analyses. Inevitably, the reviews in this book will be selective. But they highlight unanswered questions about the efficacy of commonly prescribed agents.

This book will also look towards a future in which better, more specific psychiatric drugs will be developed. When the first drugs for cancer were developed fifty years ago, their effects were unpredictable, and many patients failed to respond to them. That is more or less where we are in psychiatry today. In future decades, we can hope to have as precise a therapeutic armamentarium as most other medical specialists.

Drugs for the troubled mind have helped millions. But we must acknowledge their limitations and consider the alternatives. And that is why I have written this book.

FORCES DRIVING THE USE AND MISUSE OF DRUGS

Psychiatric drugs remain, in many respects, medical miracles. No physician could treat heart disease or cancer without modern drugs, and that is equally true for the treatment of severe mental illness. I am old enough to remember a time when psychiatrists did not have any effective drugs. Until researchers discovered pharmacotherapy for schizophrenia, bipolar disorder, and severe depression, we had little to offer patients with these diagnoses. In the course of my career, I have seen patients respond to drugs in dramatic and heartening ways. There can be little doubt that psychopharmacology has been a boon to humanity, leading to enormous progress in the treatment of disease.

But psychopharmacology is a victim of its own success. Psychiatric drugs are being over-prescribed, and applied to problems they cannot solve. Many of the agents we use today are highly effective–if prescribed in an *evidence-based* way, and given for precise indications. Unfortunately that is far from the case. Many current drugs are prescribed for *off-label* purposes, without research support for these indications.

Psychiatrists may think they know how psychiatric drugs work. The facts do not support that belief. The idea that mental disorders are the result of "chemical imbalances" in the brain (which drugs supposedly put back into balance) is an over-simplified and misleading view of a complex problem. This theory is not just wrong. It leads to a more serious "imbalance", in which clinical psychiatry has come to rely almost entirely on pharmacological treatment, to the exclusion of all other options.

For the most severely ill patients, psychiatric drugs have been a very good news story. The news has not been as good for patients with less severe symptoms. For common mental disorders, such as mild depression, drugs sometimes work, but sometimes do little more than a placebo. (As I will show, placebos do much more than most physicians think). The concept of "treatment-resistant depression" implies that all one needs to do is to prescribe the right drugs to treat complex cases. But that concept actually describes a potpourri of problems, some of which will respond to pharmacotherapy, and some of which will not.

Clinicians have been sold the myth of experts who know how to mix and match the right cocktail of medications, and that it is possible to make almost any patient better with an artful prescription. In fact, only a few drug combinations have been properly tested; the mixing of multiple agents is a largely unproven procedure. Intentions are good, but results are often bad. Practices that are not evidence-based can create more problems than they solve.

Naturally, the myth of the therapeutic cocktail has been actively encouraged by the pharmaceutical industry. These corporations earn billions from the prescription of psychiatric medications. Drug companies are not in business to promote health, but to maximize profits for their shareholders. Industry marketing is a powerful driver of prescribing practices. There is little doubt that pharmaceutical companies are misleading physicians (and patients) about the value of their products. But to be corrupted and fooled, you have to be willing. The responsibility for this situation lies squarely with practitioners and with the academic leaders of psychiatry. It is up to clinicians and key opinion leaders in the field to resist these blandishments, and make decisions based on scientific evidence.

In the modern world, large numbers of people are taking (or have taken) antidepressants or some other psychoactive drug. And that is not only the case for consenting adults. Behaviorally disturbed children are now being given complex combinations of powerful drugs. I will criticize many of these practices, which are based on very little data and a great deal of "hype". A commitment to evidence-based medicine should lead to a healthy skepticism about current practices.

While this book will be critical of the pharmaceutical industry, I fully recognize that innovative, life-saving drugs have come from that source. But these companies are not charitable organizations, and their marketing departments know how to get physicians to prescribe their products. Ultimately, the responsibility for avoiding treatments that are not evidence-based lies with practitioners.

All these problems can be placed in the larger context of medical philosophy. Physicians are trained to do their utmost for patients. This laudable goal makes us over-enthusiastic. In our zeal to cure disease, we lose sight of what drugs can and cannot do. We are too keen to treat the symptoms of mental illness, but do not understand enough about its causes.

By and large, those of us who chose psychiatry did so out of idealism. We were intensely curious about the mysteries of mental illness, and wanted to help suffering patients. But in recent years, psychiatrists have succumbed to the illusion that neuroscience can solve every problem. Treatment has vastly over-run the understanding of disease, and drugs have come to dominate management. When all one has is a hammer, everything looks like a nail.

Consumers also play a role in the misuse of drugs. Psychiatrists try to meet the perceived needs of those who seek their services. While some patients still seek psychotherapy, most now expect a prescription. As the internet makes information more readily available, some of our more sophisticated patients will request the latest drugs. This problem is not unique to psychiatry. For example, our colleagues in internal medicine tend to prescribe expensive drugs to manage hypertension, even though research shows that "golden oldies" (such as diuretics) do the job just as well. And many physicians give in to patient pressure by prescribing antibiotics for viral infections when they are not indicated.

Some psychiatric patients have an absolute need for pharmacological therapy. Yet many others do not benefit from *any* existing drugs. The underlying problem is that we do not always know what we are treating. Psychiatry is a long way from developing a scientific classification of mental illness. Diagnosis is rarely a specific guide to treatment. Ultimately, pharmacotherapy can be no more precise than our understanding of disease mechanisms. While this problem is not unique to psychiatry, we must acknowledge that our current level of knowledge leaves a great deal to be desired. In practice, we do not know who will respond to a given treatment. The result is that nonresponders tend to be treated "aggressively", leading to drug regimes that do not work and that carry a high burden of side effects. Mental illness is a complex challenge, not a simple problem in chemistry that pharmaceuticals can reverse.

Psychiatrists have been enticed and excited by a wish to cure mental illness, and by the temptation to prescribe "the latest thing". Wise physicians have always known better. To quote an aphorism attributed to Hippocrates, our true role is "to cure sometimes, to relieve often, to comfort always".

A NOTE ON NOMENCLATURE

Many psychiatric drugs are marketed using different names in the USA, Canada, UK, and on the European continent. While most practitioners refer to the drugs they prescribe by easy-to-remember trade names, this book will only use generic names.

ACKNOWLEDGMENTS

I was fortunate to have two highly knowledgeable readers, David Goldbloom and Edward Shorter, who carefully read drafts of this book and made many useful suggestions for improvement. Karl Looper and Roz Paris also helped me by reading sections of the manuscript.

This book is largely based on my experiences as a teacher of psychiatry. In a series of Journal Clubs and Evidence-Based Medicine Seminars, over the last 30 years, psychiatric residents have reviewed the literature with me. I need to acknowledge a great debt to my students – to whom this book is dedicated.

Overview

Overview

CHAPTER 1

The History of Psychopharmacology

Let us begin with a thought experiment. Imagine what it was like to treat mental illness 60 years ago. If psychiatrists in that time were honest, they would have had to admit they had few options for effective pharmacotherapy. Yet they might not have seen the situation in that light. Psychiatrists could not have known that better drugs would appear within a few years. They would concentrate on available options, and convince themselves that these agents were effective.

In 1950, if a patient was anxious or had insomnia, there were barbiturates. If a patient was depressed or complained of fatigue, there were amphetamines. These drugs, though now considered not effective, were very widely prescribed. Moreover, if patients had confidence in their physicians, whatever effects these agents had would be magnified by a placebo response.

Psychiatrists may well have thought they were helping most of their patients, and even congratulated themselves on being more advanced than their colleagues in 1890 would have been. Yet in retrospect, the only important biological therapy that has survived from 60 years ago is electroconvulsive therapy (ECT). Almost none of the other agents are prescribed for the same purposes today (although stimulants are now used to treat attention deficit hyperactivity disorder).

Now imagine the practice of psychiatry 60 years from now. Although we cannot know how much drug development will advance, it seems likely that by 2070, much more effective agents will be available than those we have today. If so, future psychiatrists could be in a position to provide more consistently effective treatments for

The Use and Misuse of Psychiatric Drugs: An Evidence-Based Critique   by Joel Paris
© 2010 John Wiley & Sons, Ltd

depression, anxiety, and psychosis. They will also probably classify these conditions in a different way, allowing them to predict treatment response from diagnosis. If future practitioners were to read about how psychiatry was practiced in the early part of the twenty-first century, they might feel just as sorry for us as we do for our predecessors from 1950.

The point is that every age retains the illusion that the tools at their disposal are effective. There is progress, but it is difficult at the time to realize the limitations of therapeutic options. Taking a historical perspective helps us to be humble about what we can and cannot do for patients.

Psychiatry has come far, but has very far to go. Developing a sense of humility about drug treatment will be the main theme of this book.

1.1 BEFORE THE REVOLUTION

Starting in the early 1950s, psychopharmacology was revolutionized. Like revolutions of all kinds, this is a story of triumph and hubris.

In the years following the Second World War, psychiatrists had few options for the effective treatment of severe mental illness. It is difficult for trainees or young psychiatrists today to imagine what psychiatric hospitals were like in those days.

I had the chance to see the problem in the late 1950s, when I was an undergraduate student in psychology at the University of Michigan. A group of us volunteered to spend weekends at the nearby Ypsilanti State Hospital, which housed over 4000 inpatients. We talked to patients, and learned a little more about them from the staff.

The wards of the hospital were full of seriously ill people who were receiving very little treatment. A stuporous catatonic stood motionless in the hallway. A paranoid schizophrenic sat in the corner writing endless notes about her delusions. A manic patient was confined to bed with cold packs. A young woman who had made a serious suicide attempt had just completed a course of ECT.

Psychotic (or severely depressed) patients could languish on wards for years – unless they were fortunate enough to go into spontaneous remission. There were few specific or effective biological treatments for them. If seriously agitated, they could be sedated with barbiturates or paraldehyde. Neuroleptics had been introduced only a few years before, and psychiatrists were just starting to use chlorpromazine in small doses.

The out-patient management of common mental disorders was equally limited. Depression and anxiety, the most frequent symptoms seen in practice, were not effectively managed with barbiturates and/or amphetamines (Shorter, 2009).

Only a few treatments from this time have survived. Insulin coma therapy had inconsistent results, and fell out of favor entirely after a controlled trial failed to demonstrate its efficacy (Ackner *et al.*, 1957). Prefrontal lobotomy, after being scandalously over-prescribed, vanished almost entirely (Valenstein, 1986). The most effective treatment in psychiatry 60 years ago was electroconvulsive therapy (ECT), which remains useful today. While ECT was over-prescribed in the past (for lack of alternatives), it is an evidence-based option that can pull patients out of psychotic depression, and provide short-term control of acute schizophrenia and mania (Shorter and Healy, 2007; Fink and Taylor, 2007).

In the absence of effective pharmacological treatment, psychotherapies held sway in certain settings, particularly private hospitals and clinics. The most prominent and prestigious method of psychological treatment, usually provided in office practice, was psychoanalysis. Even then, it was widely known that psychoanalytic therapy was expensive and yielded inconsistent results (Paris, 2005). But this was the only way most clinicians knew how to talk to their patients. Alternative methods, such as cognitive behavioral therapy, had not yet been developed.

It should not therefore be surprising that many patients failed to respond to any form of treatment. In the face of intractable disease, almost anything was worth trying. At McGill University, where I work, a long-lasting scandal ensued when massive doses of ECT were given to patients with many different problems in an attempt to "depattern" them – with the idea of removing mental patterns and starting with a blank slate (Collins, 1988). This misadventure in therapeutics can only be understood in the context of the times, when alternatives were few and when rigorous empirical testing of new therapies had not yet become standard. A revolution in drug therapy was needed. And that is exactly what happened.

1.2 BREAKTHROUGH

One of my most admired teachers was a pioneer in the development of psychiatric drugs. Heinz Lehmann (1911–1999), a refugee from Germany who practiced psychiatry in Canada, always kept up with developments in Europe. That is why he became the first physician to introduce chlorpromazine and imipramine to North America.

A few years before his death, Lehmann (1993) wrote an article entitled "*Before they called it psychopharmacology.*" Lehmann observed that the field was created from scratch over a relatively brief period. Developments then moved so rapidly that they came to be called the "psychopharmacological revolution." In the 1950s and 1960s, a remarkable series of dramatic breakthroughs occurred.

This was an age of heroic pioneers (Healy, 1998). While madness has always been with us, the discovery of the first effective drugs to treat psychosis has been described as a turning point in human history (Healy, 2008). The introduction of effective antidepressants may have been less dramatic, but there is little doubt that these drugs have helped millions. Within a few years, clinicians obtained access to a whole range of agents that could control most of the major symptoms that psychiatrists treat.

In 1952, the first-generation antipsychotics (FGAs) were introduced (Delay, Deniker and Harl, 1952). Two French psychiatrists, Jean Delay (1907–1987) and Pierre Deniker (1917–1998), studied chlorpromazine, a phenothiazine (chemically an antihistamine variant) that had been developed for anesthesia. Delay and Deniker made the discovery that chlorpromazine was specifically effective for psychotic symptoms. Two years later, in North America, Lehmann and Hanrahan (1954) confirmed its efficacy in schizophrenia.

Within a few years, FGAs dominated the treatment of psychosis. There were various phenothiazines – aliphatics, piperazines, and piperidines – but all had similar effects. One problem was that emergency treatment required a highly potent drug. That was the advantage of haloperidol, which belongs to a different chemical group (the butyrophenones). Haloperidol was used routinely for several decades as the mainstay of management for psychosis. But this agent came with a high risk for neurological side effects. And many patients found these effects sufficiently troubling that they were non-compliant.

The second breakthrough was the development of effective antidepressants. The first group to be introduced was monoamine oxidase inhibitors (MAOIs). These drugs, developed to treat tuberculosis, turned out to have more dramatic effects on mood. However MAOIs have many problematic side effects, and some have since been withdrawn (Healy, 2008). Today they are rarely used for first-line therapy.

The second group of antidepressants had a more enduring impact. The tricyclics (another chemical variant of antihistamines) remain an important (but currently less often used) part of our armamentarium. The Swiss psychiatrist Roland Kuhn (1912–2005) was the first to report on the effectiveness of imipramine (Kuhn, 1958). This agent was (and is) particularly useful for severe depression. Chapter 6 will examine whether it has been superceded by any of the alternatives introduced since. Within a few years after its introduction, imipramine (and several other tricylics) were very widely prescribed, leading to a decline in the use of ECT (Shorter and Healy, 2007).

The third major development of the 1950s was the introduction of anxiolytics (originally called "tranquilizers"). The first agent to be introduced, meprobamate, was widely prescribed for a number of years, but fell out of favor. This was partly out of concern about side effects, but mainly because it was replaced by the benzodiazepines (Shorter, 2009; Tone, 2008).

Like many other drugs in medicine, "benzos" are derived from chemical dyes. A pharmacologist, Leo Sternbach (1908–2005) noticed that these molecules made him drowsy, and went on to develop both chlordiazepoxide and diazepam. These drugs (and their variants) continue to be in standard use today.

Another major breakthrough of the psychopharmacological revolution took place some years later – in the late 1960s, when lithium was introduced for the treatment of mania. An Australian psychiatrist, John Cade (1912–1980), made the first observations on the effectiveness of lithium (Cade, 1949). However concern about side effects on the heart discouraged its wider use. Lithium was rediscovered and systematically investigated by the Danish psychiatrist Mogens Schou (1918–2005). This research (Baastrup and Schou, 1967) led to its wide use, both for acute mania and for the prevention of relapse in both phases of bipolar disorder.

Thus by 1970, psychiatrists could choose from a pharmacological armamentarium that included antipsychotics, antidepressants, anxiolytics, and antimanics. That toolbox (along with ECT) was almost as good as what we have 40 years later. With a few modern additions, these groups of drugs are the backbone of management for most severe mental disorders today.

In the modern world, we tend to assume that progress is inevitable, and that one breakthrough will inevitably follow another. In the age of neuroscience, research on the brain has been expected to produce rapid and dramatic progress that can be applied to clinical problems. Many of us have come to believe that when it comes to drugs, newer is better.

In fact, psychopharmacology is not much more effective than it was in 1970. New drugs have been introduced with fewer (or different) side effects. But we are not doing that much more for patients. We are much like internists who treat hypertension with expensive ACE inhibitors instead of diuretics. Psychiatry can be practiced effectively using drugs that were available 40 years ago.

Moreover, drug development has been more the result of luck than of planning (Healy, 2002). Phenothiazines were originally introduced for sedation, and their antipsychotic effects came as a surprise. Tricyclics are chemically similar to phenothiazines, and were originally thought to have the same indications – their efficacy in depression came as another surprise. Lithium, originally developed as a cardiac drug, turned out to have much more useful antimanic effects.

Moreover, breakthroughs mostly arose from careful clinical observation. The effectiveness of new drugs was only confirmed later by randomized controlled trials. This was an era when formal research in medical science was relatively undeveloped. While standards for evidence-base medicine were primitive, talented psychiatrists who were willing to try out new agents could make a real mark on their field.

Moreover, pharmacological treatments for mental illness revolutionized practice. Within a few years, older drugs were forgotten, and resistance from older clinicians melted away. A large body of research confirmed that there was no substitute for the new drugs. For example, neuroleptics were definitively shown by a controlled trial to be superior to either talking therapies or ECT in schizophrenia (May,

1968). Tricyclics were found to be superior to either cognitive or interpersonal psychotherapy for severe depression (Elkin *et al.*, 1989). Lithium was (and remains) superior to any alternative for preventing relapse of bipolar disorder (Goodwin and Jamieson, 2007).

It became widely accepted in psychiatry that patients with mental illness usually need drugs. Expertise in prescription became central to the identity of psychiatrists (Paris, 2008a). In the USA, a failure to prescribe antidepressants for severe depressive illness (in a patient named Raphael Osheroff, himself a physician) became the basis of a famous lawsuit (Klerman, 1990). After the Osheroff case, fewer psychiatrists were willing to treat depression with talking therapy alone.

The period from 1952 to 1970 was the golden age of psychopharmacology, a time of continuous triumph for psychiatric drugs. Mental hospitals emptied out and closed entirely – largely due to drug therapy (but also to better community psychiatry). Ypsilanti State, the enormous hospital that I had visited in 1958, closed in 1992, and has since been demolished.

1.3 AFTER THE REVOLUTION

Revolutions tend to be followed by periods of consolidation. Over the last 40 years, no change of the same magnitude occurred in psychopharmacology. Instead, atypical (second-generation) antipsychotics replaced typicals, specific serotonin reuptake inhibitors replaced tricyclics, and anticonvulsant mood stabilizers partially replaced lithium. While we now had more alternatives, the newer drugs were not always better than older ones (which younger psychiatrists no longer knew how to use). The main advantage was that some of the newer agents (e.g., SSRIs) had fewer side effects than their predecessors and required less careful titration of dose.

For these reasons non-psychiatric physicians became more comfortable with prescribing these agents. Thus, drugs to treat mental symptoms became ubiquitous in general medicine. Today, primary care physicians (and psychologists) treat most patients with less severe mental disorders, while specialists in psychiatry tend to see treatment-resistant cases.

Another caveat about the triumph of psychopharmacology is that in spite of a greater ability to control symptoms, psychiatrists have not been able to *cure* most of the conditions they treat. There is a big difference between symptomatic improvement and full remission.

For example, in spite of the efficacy of neuroleptics for acute psychotic symptoms, schizophrenia remains a chronic and disabling disease. And in spite of the efficacy of lithium for acute manic symptoms and for prevention of relapses, bipolar disorder remains a serious clinical problem, for which no definitive therapy has emerged. Finally, in spite of the efficacy of antidepressants, many depressions remain treatment-resistant and/or chronic (Fava and Rush, 2006).

In summary, after a period of breakthrough and revolution, progress in the pharmacological treatment of mental illness has been quite slow. The amount and quality of research has greatly increased, and there is little doubt that we know more about how the brain works. However, there is no reason to believe treatment has advanced since the 1970s. In the last decade or so, no drugs have been introduced that even remotely constitute a therapeutic breakthrough.

Even so, there has been a good deal of "hype" around newer drugs. That is mainly due to aggressive industry marketing, as well as the assumption that whatever is newer must be better. In reality, the golden age is behind us. By a combination of brilliance and luck, researchers found ways to manage patients for whom no useful treatment had been available. The last 40 years have been more of a slog than a breakthrough.

We could be lucky again. But I am inclined to believe that future progress in psychopharmacology needs to wait for a better understanding of the causes of mental illness. We still do not know why patients develop schizophrenia, mania, or depression, or whether these conditions need to be classified in a new way (Tyrer and Kendall, 2009). We also do not know how the drugs we are currently using actually work.

The good news is, as the next chapter will show, that we now apply much higher standards for the assessment of new drugs. It is no longer sufficient to try out an agent on 10 or 20 patients and observe results. We have entered an era of evidence-based psychiatry. In the long run, drug treatment is bound to benefit from a scientific approach.

CHAPTER 2

The Science of Psychopharmacology

2.1 DRUGS, MIND, AND BRAIN

Many lectures in psychopharmacology use slides with pictures of a synapse, purportedly showing how drugs affect neurotransmission. Psychiatrists like to believe that the drugs they prescribe have precise, scientifically proven effects on the brain. But the fact is that while we understand what these agents can do, we do not know how they work. Psychiatric drugs were discovered by serendipity, and their mechanism of action is still largely a mystery.

Actually this is not an unusual situation in medicine. The precise action of digitalis was established two centuries after the Scottish physician William Withering (1741–1799) observed that an extract of the common plant purple foxglove was useful for "dropsy." The mechanism of effect of penicillin on bacteria was unknown for decades after its famous (and accidental) discovery by the Scottish pharmacologist Alexander Fleming (1881–1955).

Yet even if other specialists may also be groping in the dark, there is a profound disconnect between psychiatry and the rest of medicine. Psychiatrists study and treat diseases of the mind. Mental activity is a function of neurons, and to understand psychiatric drugs, we need to find out in some detail how the brain works. That is a project that will take centuries, not decades.

The brain is the most fantastically complicated structure in all of nature. It is estimated to have 100 billion neurons (and an even larger number of glial cells), with a total number of synapses that has been conservatively estimated at 60 *trillion* (Shepherd, 1998). To put these numbers in perspective, an average galaxy contains "only" 100 billion stars.

Moreover, each part of the brain has multiple functions and participates in multiple circuits. We know of about 100 neurotransmitters. But they do not always have the same effect, since all neurons have multiple receptor proteins that bind uniquely to these chemical messengers. Thus each neurotransmitter can perform a different function, depending on anatomical location and type of receptor.

We are looking at a level of complexity that dwarfs the physiology of any other organ in the body, such as the heart, or the kidney. It is no wonder that science is only just beginning to understand the brain. Or that psychopharmacology is in the earliest stages of its development.

2.2 NEUROTRANSMITTERS

Drugs are chemicals, and their main mechanism of action on the brain lies in chemistry. These agents attach themselves to receptors, either blocking or enhancing the role of neurotransmitters. Yet most drugs act on more than one receptor. As Healy (2009) neatly puts it, psychiatric drugs are cocktails, not magic bullets.

The most influential theory of how drugs work in the brain is based on their effects on neurotransmitters at the synapse. The essential concept is that mental disorders occur when transmitters are either too active or insufficiently active, and/or when there is an imbalance between the activity of different transmitters. This scenario is popularly referred to (especially by patients) as a "chemical imbalance." Drugs, which act on receptors, are supposed to restore these balances. Yet there is *no* convincing evidence that this hypothesis is in any way valid (Valenstein, 2005; Healy, 2009; Kirsch, 2009). The relationship of neurochemistry to behavior is much too complex for such an explanation.

Most research on neurotransmitters has concerned small molecules such as: acetylcholine (ACh), norepinephrine (NE), dopamine (DA), serotonin (5-HT), melatonin, histamine, glutamate, gamma aminobutyric acid (GABA), aspartate, and glycine. The most widely distributed neurotransmitters in the brain are glutamate – which is excitatory, and gamma-aminobutyric acid (GABA) – which is inhibitory. Over 90% of all brain synapses use one or another of these two messengers. Yet surprisingly, research on the activity of glutamate and GABA is a relatively recently development. Their central role in neurotransmission was hardly known until a few years ago. (This fact should give us pause as to how well, even now, we understand neurochemistry.)

Glutamate acts on the NMDA (N-methyl D-aspartate) receptor. In recent years it has been suggested that abnormalities in its transmission might be related to schizophrenia (Lisman *et al.*, 2008). Thus far, that theory has not led to the development of any new antipsychotic drugs. In contrast, drugs that have effects on GABA produce changes that closely correspond to its inhibitory function. Alcohol, sedatives, and benzodiazepines all target these receptors. This seems to be the one aspect of neurotransmission in which chemistry has specific effects.

The monoamines – dopamine, NE, and 5-HT – have crucial modulating effects on neurons that use glutamate or GABA. Many drugs used in contemporary practice have primary effects on neurotransmitters acting on circuits using these molecules. However, the mechanisms are very complex, and effects further down the chain of proteins ("second or third messengers") vastly complicate the relationship between drug actions and neural activity.

The human mind loves simplicity. Many theories have suggested that abnormalities in monoamine receptors are directly associated with mental disorders. The dopaminergic model of schizophrenia was highly influential for decades. That theory was based on the observation that most antipsychotics have DA-antagonistic effects, and that hyperactive dopaminergic signals could be responsible for schizophrenic symptoms (Seeman *et al.*, 1976). More specifically, it was hypothesized that overactivity of these receptors – a specific group (D2), or an excessive number of dopamine receptors – could be of key importance in psychosis (Seeman and Kapur, 2000).

However a great deal of evidence has challenged this theory (Moncrieff, 2009). For example, atypical neuroleptics, which have much less effect on dopamine receptors, are as effective for psychotic symptoms as typicals. After a generation of research, most researchers agree that the dopamine theory of schizophrenia was greatly oversim-plified (Tost, Alam, and Meyer-Lindenberg, 2009).

The monoamine theory of depression has also been extremely in-fluential (Heninger et al., 1996). It proposed that the underlying bio-logical basis for lowered mood is a deficiency of central noradrenergic and/or serotonergic systems. Targeting these systems with an antide-pressant would therefore restore neural function.

There are many problems with this theory. The most obvious is that antidepressants do not consistently lead to remission of de-pression (see Chapter 6). Of course, treatments based on correct etiological theories may not prove to be effective in practice. But 30 years or more after the hypothesis was first proposed, there is no research evidence for any monoamine deficiency in depressed patients (Valenstein, 1998). While antidepressants certainly have an effect on monoamines, as shown by both human and animal studies, we cannot conclude that this provides an explanation of their effects on the brain (Healy, 2009). Thus, while monoamines undoubtedly play an impor-tant modulatory role on neurotransmission, their activity has not, by itself, provided an explanation of depressed mood (Heninger *et al.*, 1996).

There is actually stronger evidence supporting a role for serotonin in conditions that are *not* mood disorders. Antidepressants, particu-larly those that are serotonergic, have anxiolytic effects, while sero-tonergic antidepressants have relatively specific effects on the symp-toms of obsessive-compulsive disorder (see Chapter 6). And although impulsive symptoms do not necessarily respond to antidepressants, there is robust evidence that patients with substance abuse and impul-sive aggression have abnormalities of the central serotonergic system (Moeller *et al.*, 2001). And these relationships are stronger than any links between serotonin and mood.

The lesson to be learned is that neurotransmitters serve a variety of functions in the brain. They are not related to a single syndrome or disorder. The brain is not a chemical soup. You cannot study drug actions without considering neurocircuitry. For this reason, we are unlikely to ever find a drug that treats a mental illness by specifically targeting a single molecule or molecular pathway.

Alternative explanations of drug action that do not primarily involve neurotransmitters are also possible. For example, it has been suggested that antidepressants may stimulate the development of new synapses, and there is some evidence from animal studies (Zhou *et al.*, 2006) that SSRIs increase brain-derived neurotrophic factor (BDNF), a protein that promotes neural growth. But we do not know whether this process occurs in humans, or whether it can explain how antidepressants work in the brain.

In summary, while neuroscience research is exciting, it has been greatly over-hyped. We are in love with beautiful (but artificially) colored pictures provided by brain scans, and by diagrams purporting to show how drugs affect neurons and synapses. The reality is that while researchers have learned a great deal about the brain in recent decades, clinical applications remain a promise, not a reality.

Consider, for example, how neuroscience has progressed in localizing brain functions. Today, we know much more about the relationship of the limbic system, particularly the amygdala, with abnormalities of emotion, as well as the relationship between specific cortical sites and abnormalities in cognition, planning, and decision making (Miller and Cohen, 2001). But localization at the cortical level is far from precise: except for motor and sensory cortex, there is no such thing as a one-to-one correspondence between any one region and any specific function. You cannot predict thoughts, emotions, or behavior on the basis of what area of the brain "lights up" on a scan. These circuits are widespread, involving interactions between many neurons in many different regions (recall those 60 trillion synapses).

It is also questionable whether mental activity can *ever* be, even in principle, fully explained at a neuronal level. Philosophically, the mind is a complex and "emergent" phenomenon that cannot be reduced to processes at the level of cells or synapses (Paris, 2009; Gold, 2009). I am not, of course, advocating dualism, or suggesting that mind can exist independent of brain. The point is that complex systems cannot be reduced to and explained by their components.

For this reason, proposals that psychiatry should eventually become a branch of "clinical neuroscience" (Insel and Quirion, 2005) are, at best, naïve. To understand the mind and mental illness, we need to build bridges between neuroscience and psychology – a discipline that studies mental processes on their own terms.

The belief that neuroscience will lead to drug development is another promise that has not been fulfilled. This hope is based on an oversimplification. Pharmacological agents have widespread and diffuse effects and do not target one brain system. Drugs will always be relatively blunt instruments. (Again, think cocktails, not magic bullets.)

Another hope is that understanding the genome will lead to gene-based drug development that will make pharmacotherapy more specific (Rane, 2001). This idea is questionable – for similar reasons. While most human genes are active in the brain (Andreasen, 2001), there is no direct correspondence between any specific genetic locus and brain structures or functions. Mental processes and behaviors are influenced by *many* genes – each of which can be turned on or turned off by epigenetic mechanisms. It is therefore not surprising that expectations that specific genes might be discovered that would account for the development of any mental disorder have not been met (Kendler, 2005).

One of the main reasons for lack of progress in applying neuroscience to psychiatry is the "phenotype problem." In other words, you can't define a disease properly, you won't be able to establish genetic relationships. Mental disorders are not true phenotypes, but provisional classifications of observable phenomena. What needs to be discovered are the pathological pathways or "endophenotypes" that underlie observable symptoms (Braff *et al.*, 2007).

The main reason why molecular genetics has not helped to develop new drug therapies is that mental disorders, like most medical conditions, are rooted in "complex inheritance," that is, psychopathological mechanisms that reflect the interaction of multiple genes, each of which has a relatively small effect (Kendler and Prescott, 2006). That is why understanding genetic mechanisms may not lead to cures. Even in a disease like cystic fibrosis, where one major recessive allele has been discovered, research has not led to effective therapy (Griesenbach *et al.*, 2006).

Finally, genes do not act independently of the environment context and cannot be understood outside that context. The new science of *epigenomics* shows how genes are activated or inactivated by the environment (Beck and Olek, 2003; Rutter, 2006). Some of the molecular switches (methyl groups and histones) that mediate epigenetic mechanisms can be passed on to the next generation (Sng and Meaney, 2009).

Some widely quoted research on prospectively followed community cohorts has suggested that genetic vulnerability may not be pathogenic at all unless it interacts with environmental stressors (Caspi *et al.*, 2002, 2003). But while the principle may be correct, the hypothesized relationship between variants in the serotonin transporter gene, environmental stressors and depression has actually not been confirmed, as shown by a recent meta-analysis (Risch *et al.*, 2009). Again, the problem is that one can predict very little from a single gene. This kind of research needs to be conducted by looking at multiple alleles.

In summary, the relationship of neurotransmitters to behavior is in no way simple or linear. That is why changing the activity of receptors and transmitters at the synapse does not produce predictable consequences. Moreover, biological mechanisms can be changed by interventions at a psychological level. No matter how useful drugs are as tools for the treatment of mental disorders, psychiatric treatment will never be *entirely* based on pharmacology.

2.3 DIAGNOSES AND SYMPTOMS

In spite of these caveats, future advances in psychopharmacology could benefit from the identification of more precise neurobiological mechanisms behind disease. But the disorders described in manuals like the American Psychiatric Association's "DSM" series are *not* diseases. They are symptomatic presentations, that is, surface manifestations of hidden processes. Once understood, underlying *endophenotypes* might provide more specific targets for intervention. But we currently lack the knowledge to do so. Using drugs to treat observable symptoms rather than disease processes is something of a shot in the dark (even if it sometimes works).

Like all physicians, psychiatrists take histories, observe symptoms, and use these data to make diagnoses. But unlike many other specialists, they have no access to laboratory findings that could shed light on psychopathological processes. To develop a better system of categorizing illness, they will need to identify biological markers that point to specific disease mechanisms. At this point, diagnosis in psychiatry is, at best, a rough-and-ready tool.

In general medicine, even though some conditions are better understood than others, more illness categories are based on an understanding of etiology and pathogenesis. Diseases like myocardial infarction or stroke have known mechanisms, specific and observable clinical effects, and can be diagnosed with the help of laboratory tests and/or imaging methods.

The situation in psychiatry is different. We pride ourselves on obtaining detailed histories and making careful observations of mental states. This "phenomenological" approach provides much useful information (and we are right to be proud of these clinical skills). But psychiatrists are not yet in a position to "examine" the brain.

Signs and symptoms do not define diseases. When symptoms consistently appear together, that constitutes a *syndrome*. Examples in medicine include anemia, jaundice, chest pain, or peripheral edema. All of these phenomena can reflect entirely different pathological processes. None are valid categories of disease.

It is the absence of knowledge as to what causes and maintains disease processes that has forced psychiatric diagnosis, thus far, to be almost exclusively based on phenomenology. It is certainly better to rely on what you can see than to impose an incorrect theory. Both DSM-IV-TR (American Psychiatric Association, 2000) and ICD-10 (World Health Organization, 1992) adopted the phenomenological approach. (Actually they had no choice.) The DSM manual describes the clinical features of each category and then defines an algorithm, in which one makes a diagnosis based on a specific number of signs and symptoms (only some of which are absolutely required). ICD is similar, but asks clinicians whether the patient's clinical picture approximates a prototype.

But as recognized by the pioneer psychiatrist Emil Kraepelin (1856–1928), such methods can only be a provisional way of developing valid illness categories. The greatest advances in medicine have been based on a detailed understanding of pathogenesis and etiology.

Thus psychiatrists should not fall into the trap of believing that categories such as "major depression" are diseases, in the same sense as hepatitis A or multiple sclerosis. As we will see, that idea has led to a widespread and inappropriate use of drug therapy.

Diagnosis is nonetheless essential for practice. At the very least, it provides a common language for physicians. When we say a patient has schizophrenia, bipolar disorder, or anorexia nervosa, we are conveying important information. But in the long run, these categories may or may not turn out to be either homogeneous or valid.

A truly scientific classification needs to describe disorders with a specific etiology and pathogenesis. That is very far from the case in psychiatry. Schizophrenia is as mysterious as it has always been – it could be one disease or several. Bipolar disorder in its classical form seems to constitute a medical illness, but its boundaries remain unclear. Major depression is highly heterogeneous, making it a thorny category with a relatively unpredictable response to treatment. These problems occur in other specialties, particularly when illness mechanisms are not yet understood. But they are more severe in psychiatry.

Attempts to cut this Gordian knot have thus far been unsuccessful. Many years ago, the American psychiatrist Donald Klein proposed that response to drugs could be used as a marker for unique pathogenetic pathways. In this way, diagnosis would be based on "pharmacological dissection." This intriguing concept was used by Klein (1978) to define the difference between a panic attack (which responds to antidepressants) and accompanying anticipatory anxiety (which does not). However, pharmacological dissection has thus far provided little insight into pathological mechanisms.

The problem, once again, is that psychiatric drugs show more overlap than specificity in relation to diagnostic categories (Healy, 2009). Many agents work for reasons that remain unknown. These mechanisms have not helped us to develop a valid diagnostic system rooted in neuroscience.

Actually, most of the agents used in psychiatry are more like Aspirin (which has non-specific effects on fever and inflammation) than like antibiotics (which have specific effects on bacterial infections). They target symptoms, not disorders.

I have noted how much of the psychopharmacology literature gives the impression that our knowledge of how drugs target receptors establishes some degree of specificity for their action on the brain. But as Healy (2009) rightly observes, the fact that Aspirin acts on the prostaglandin system does not prove that prostaglandins are at fault when a patient feels pain.

Drug response may never be the basis for a valid diagnostic system. For example, antipsychotic drugs reduce paranoid thinking and hallucinations in a wide variety of conditions – including schizophrenia, mania, psychotic depression, organic brain syndromes, and personality disorders. Moreover, antipsychotics, in spite of their name, do not lead to full remission in any of the diseases in which psychotic symptoms occur. Similarly, antidepressants have broad effects on many symptoms, and do not define the nature of depression.

2.4 CLINICAL JUDGMENT

Everyone today agrees that the practice of medicine should be evidence-based. Even so, different physicians can offer quite different treatments. Most practitioners make choices that depend on their clinical judgment and experience. As a physician who is getting on in years, I would not want to dismiss the value of experience. In medicine, the charismatic and silver-haired practitioner of many years standing still carries a fair degree of clout. But relying on clinical judgment can sometimes lead us to make irrational choices. (It has been said that clinical experience could be defined as repeating the same mistake with increasing levels of confidence.)

Groopman (2007) has described some of the mistakes in medical practice that arise from cognitive biases. First and foremost, pre-existing ideas influence our judgments, and lead to mistaken confirmation of previous beliefs. For example, practice always has a *selection bias*, so that clinicians tend to be impressed with the most severe cases they see, rather than considering the characteristics of broader patient populations.

A second set of problems derive from an *availability bias*. We try to explain clinical phenomena, and attribute them to something readily at hand, such as a prescription, particularly the last one we wrote. This is an example of a famous fallacy, "Post hoc ergo propter hoc" (after this, therefore because of this).

There can be many reasons why patients get better (or worse). Some arise from environmental changes that may or not be observed or monitored. Others arise from the natural fluctuation of disease processes (which is why many drugs seem to work for a while, and then seem to "poop out"). Also, a patient may be admitted to a ward, or enter a new program that raises their hopes and expectations. In each of these cases, if change is attributed to a drug, both patient and physician may be convinced that the recently prescribed agent is absolutely essential.

To correct these errors, there is no substitute for systematic research. Science prevents us from jumping to false conclusions. It converts observations into numbers and puts hypotheses to the test.

2.5   EVIDENCE-BASED PSYCHIATRY

The movement to make clinical practice more scientific is called evidence-based medicine (EBM). The Scottish physician Archie Cochrane (1909–1988) was one of the main founders of EBM. Cochrane lived an adventurous life. After his medical training, he underwent psychoanalysis in Vienna, fought in the Spanish Civil War, and spent the Second World War as a German prisoner. After the war, Cochrane became an academic physician in Cardiff, specializing in the treatment of tuberculosis. (This was the time when strepto-mycin treatment for TB became the subject of the first clinical trial in medicine, for which the Russian-American microbiologist Selman Waksman won a Nobel Prize.)

Cochrane (1972) always emphasized that given limited resources, managing health care always requires choices, and that these choices should, in principle, be based on evidence from randomized controlled trials (RCTs). These ideas eventually lead to the establishment of the Cochrane Library database of systematic reviews, the UK Cochrane Centre at Oxford, and the international Cochrane Collaboration. More than 20 years after his death, the name *Cochrane* remains associated with skeptical, thorough, and demanding reviews of almost every kind of medical treatment.

The movement benefited from other pioneers. EBM is now mainly centered in Oxford, but a Canadian group located at McMaster University in Hamilton, Ontario, played an important role.

EBM gradually became a dominant force in the assessment of medical care. An article in the *Journal of the American Medical Association* (Evidence-Based Medicine Group, 1992) describing the principles of EBM was one of the most highly cited papers in the history of medicine.

Prescribing on the basis of solid empirical data lies at the core of evidence-based practice. In the last few decades, at the same time as useful psychiatric drugs were being developed, medical treatment as a whole has undergone a revolution.

While therapy should be based, as much as possible, on the findings of scientific research, for lack of sufficient data, many (if not most) clinical decisions that physicians make cannot be evidence-based. Another problem is that physicians may not be aware of what science has found, in which case research has little effect on practice.

We are still in a better situation than in the past, when *all* choices of medical treatment were based on tradition and clinical lore. In the late nineteenth and early twentieth century, academic physicians such as William Osler (1856–1919) began to advocate scientific medicine. But the data were much too thin to provide enough solid guidance, and most clinical decisions still had to depend almost entirely on experience.

For these reasons, practice has been more of a craft than a science. In the past, medical students were taught to revere their teachers and follow their accumulated wisdom. But even the most extensive clinical experience can lead to wrong conclusions. For example, when I was a student, surgeons treating breast cancer insisted on carrying out radical mastectomies, even when the evidence showed that local excision of a tumor was equally effective.

Let us examine how EBM principles apply to pharmacotherapy. EBM describes several levels of evidence that can be used to support the efficacy of any treatment. The highest level consists of multiple sources of evidence pointing in the same direction, as in a meta-analysis. It is always better to draw on multiple sources of data than to depend on any one study. I teach my students never to change their practice based on a single journal article, no matter how impressive it seems. As shown by Ioannidis (2005), most published research findings turn out to be false.

However meta-analyses have an Achilles heel – combining a large number of studies, each of which has made use of a different sample, may or may not yield clinically relevant results. Meta-analyses are supposed to compensate for the faults of individual studies by using pooled data. But combining data based on small unrepresentative samples can lead to misleading results. In addition, meta-analyses may combine data on many different types of treatment and/or many different groups of patients (Hatala *et al.*, 2005). So even the highest standard of evidence may not always be good enough.

Next in the hierarchy comes high quality RCTs. The presence of a control group and the blinding of raters to treatment provide a protection against seeing only what we want to see. If an RCT is designed properly, then any differences between treated patients and controls should be due to the agent under study.

Lower down on the hierarchy are single-blinded trials, open trials, and the humble case report. While drugs have sometimes been discovered from such approaches, none of these methods can really be trusted. The case report (or series of case reports) constitutes the lowest level of evidence. Today this approach can only be defended if one is studying a rare disease, or as a prelude to carrying out a formal clinical trial.

While RCTs are usually the best way to test drugs, they suffer from important limitations. First, while it is very important that the sample be representative of real-world medicine, that is hardly ever the case. Patients who sign up for clinical trials may be less sick, motivated by a wish to earn money, or have a history of not having not benefited from other forms of treatment (Westen and Morrison, 2001). Moreover, not every patient will agree to enter a trial and to be randomized. Many will insist on getting what they believe to be the "best" treatment. Of crucial importance, many drug trials are conducted on volunteers who answer advertisements – a group in no way representative of clinical reality.

Another reason why RCTs are unrepresentative is that the sickest patients can be excluded by design. For example, subjects in depression trials typically have mild symptoms, and may therefore not respond as well to drugs (Parker, 2009). In some medical specialties, such as oncology, trials tend to be conducted on the sickest patients (who have little to lose). But in psychiatry, patients in clinical trials are usually less ill, with fewer "comorbid" conditions. Many RCT protocols have exclusions for subjects with common comorbidities (such as substance abuse), seriously under-representing the patients with complex pathology that clinicians see every day.

In clinical research, *sampling is everything*. For this reason, even meta-analyses, if they combine the results of many studies, each of which has an unrepresentative sample, may not produce results that are relevant to practice.

Still another problem is that patients in RCTs need to complete a clinical trial. In reality, many do not – and these less compliant patients can closely resemble cases seen in practice. For that reason, results need to be analyzed on an "intention to treat" basis, which means including everyone who started the trial, even if (and especially if) they dropped out early). This important step is not always carried out.

One of the most pervasive problems for RCTs is low power. Too many studies have just enough subjects to obtain significance at $p < 0.05$. But findings with small sample sizes may not be replicable. Results in selected subjects cannot be assumed to be generalizable to the real world of practice.

Moreover, statistical significance does not translate into clinical significance. Many RCTs will report positive results if patients move a few points on a rating scale. Again reaching $p < 0.05$ is seen as a gold standard. But even when patients are somewhat improved, they may remain ill. *Remission* of illness is a more demanding standard than clinical improvement. It has only recently been used on a regular basis in clinical research.

Another problem is that most clinical trials are of short duration. Many if not most mental disorders are chronic, and drugs often need to be taken for years. Yet very few RCTs last for more than three months. As later chapters will show, the lack of a longer follow-up can make the clinical application of research very doubtful.

Also, newer drugs are rarely placed in head-to-head comparisons with existing agents. Placebo comparisons are necessary but lower the bar and make it easier to show an effect. They do not tell you whether a new drug is better than an old one.

Finally, RCTs are very expensive. For that reason, most are paid for by manufacturers, and are biased in favor of positive results. Moreover, many badly needed studies have never been conducted. As Chapter 3 will show, one should not trust industry-funded RCTs.

For all these reasons, RCTs, while still the best way to test drugs, do not answer some of the most pressing questions that face clinicians. Thus, in addition to *efficacy* studies (randomized controlled trials), researchers need to conduct *effectiveness* studies, in which a treatment's effect is measured in an unselected clinical population (Summerfelt and Meltzer, 1998). These two options are complementary, since RCTs are controlled but tend to use highly selected, non-generalizable samples, while effectiveness studies lack comparisons of drugs to no treatment. Thus while effectiveness studies, which lack placebo controls, cannot determine whether a drug really works, they are a necessary second step to see whether efficacy data translates into the real world of practice. Unfortunately, this type of research is also expensive (and rare).

Again, keep in mind that single studies of any kind, no matter how well designed, may or may not be replicated. Every physician needs to keep this point in mind before being impressed by "the latest thing." Before trying out new drugs, it may be wise to wait until they have been around for a few years and have been more widely tested.

In the world of EBM, it is agreed that the highest quality of evidence comes from systematic reviews, meta-analyses of multiple RCTs, or multiple meta-analyses that all lead to the same conclusion. In spite of all the problems discussed above, that is the kind of data that should guide practice. But since it is not possible to practice medicine *entirely* on the basis of research, one has to leave some room for less demanding levels of evidence. If all one has to go on is uncontrolled open trials, is weak data better than none at all? I would say no. Good journals almost never publish such papers. If you seriously want to determine efficacy, why not carry out an RCT?

The EBM movement is only the beginning of a long journey for medicine. Treatment decisions still have to be made on individual patients, not populations (Groopman, 2007). Yet no matter how experienced the physician, there is more likelihood of error if clinical decisions are made without support from research. Physicians should be humble about what they do not know, and not cover over their ignorance with false certainty.

2.6 CONDUCTING CLINICAL TRIALS

While many drugs in medicine can be tested on animals, doing so is not feasible in psychiatry. Animals have different mental capacities, and do not suffer from the same illnesses as we do. Major mental disorders such as schizophrenia and mania occur exclusively in humans. We can test for drug safety in other species, but not for efficacy.

The best case for an animal model is substance abuse, since other species can be made physiologically dependent on alcohol or drugs (Miller and Carroll, 2006). There have also been animal models of depression (Deussing, 2006), although their application to clinical work is uncertain. Researchers in mood disorders can study how long it takes a rat to give up swimming when confined to a small pool, and measure the effects of antidepressants on that behavior (Norman and McGrath, 2000). But while a "learned helplessness" model is an *analog* of depression, it is not the same phenomenon. Some of the most severe depressions have little to do with disappointment or defeat, but come "out of the blue" without any obvious trigger.

Thus psychiatric drugs need to be researched in human subjects. There is a standard protocol for conducting clinical trials. To protect subjects from unknown effects, they are traditionally carried out in several "phases." In phase 1, safety and tolerability are examined by administering the drug to a small group of healthy volunteers. In phase II, the drug is systematically assessed in a larger sample of people who have the disorder for which the drug is being evaluated. Phase III consists (ideally) of multi-centered RCTs to examine efficacy of the drug for specific target symptoms. Phase IV involves post-marketing surveillance after a drug is approved.

To establish efficacy, drugs are compared either to an existing "gold standard" treatment, or (when no treatment is known to be effective) to a placebo. But even when an established therapy exists, there is a continuing controversy as to whether placebo trials are ethical (Emanuel and Miller, 2001). If you don't know whether a drug will work at all, you should compare it to no treatment. The question is whether it is ethical to deny patients in a trial the benefit of an established therapy for their symptoms.

By and large, new drugs tend to look better when compared to inactive treatments. But when drugs are submitted for approval, the fact that they are better than placebo does not tell you whether they are better than existing alternatives. When a comparative trial is carried out, without a placebo arm, a new treatment might appear to have similar efficacy to a standard treatment, yet be no better than a placebo

(Young and Annable, 2002). Drug trials would therefore benefit from comparisons both to existing treatment *and* to placebo.

Another set of problems concerns the statistical analysis of results. As discussed earlier, many outcome measures in RCTs represent a partial improvement rather than a remission. Moreover, clinical trials need to do more than support yes-no decisions about efficacy. Classical tests of statistical significance in research tell you *whether* a drug is better than placebo (again, at the $p < 0.05$ level), but not by *how much*. For this reason, research in medicine and the social sciences has turned increasingly to the measurement of *effect sizes* (Montori *et al.*, 2004). Sometimes clinical trials describe effects that are statistically significant but not *clinically* significant. (The patient has fewer symptoms but remains ill.) Effect sizes tell you how much patients have moved from their baseline in standard deviation units. Small changes emerge from many trials. But if you observe effect sizes of at least half a standard deviation, you are probably looking at clinically significant change.

To address quantitative issues in clinical trials, it is useful to apply some measures derived from epidemiological research. For example, one can examine whether a drug reduces *absolute risk* for developing a symptom, that is, a *difference* between treated groups and controls, as well as *relative risk*, that is, a *ratio* between treated groups and controls (Barratt *et al.*, 2004). By and large, absolute risk is a better measure, since relative risk tends to exaggerate effectiveness (many clinical trials have reported small misleadingly differences in this way). For example, a treatment that reduces your chance of a stroke by 50% sounds good; however that is a relative risk reduction. If the risk of stroke only decreases from 2 in 10,000 to 1 in 10,000, then your absolute risk reduction is not very impressive. In such cases, the significance of side effects associated with a relative reduction may loom larger.

Another important statistic is the Number Needed to Treat (NNT), that is, the number of patients who need to be treated in order to prevent one additional negative outcome (McAlister, 2008). This is the inverse of an absolute risk reduction associated with a drug treatment. Such information helps determine whether a drug is cost-effective. A related statistic is the Number Needed to Harm (NNH), that is, the number of patients exposed to a drug that will cause harm in at least one case. That information tells you if the benefit from an agent is greater than its risk.

With these tools in hand, the results of clinical trials can be measured in a more precise way than they were in the past. Keeping these principles in mind can help us to be skeptical of industry-sponsored claims for psychiatric drugs.

2.7 PLACEBO EFFECTS

There is another reason why RCTs are necessary – the enormous power of a placebo. These effects are like the proverbial elephant in the room – one ignores them at one's peril.

Although all physicians know about placebo effects, they consistently underestimate them. A large body of research shows that placebos are powerful agents, reducing symptoms in a wide variety of medical conditions (Benedetti, 2008).

We are all familiar with the idea that an inert agent can be effective if a patient expects it to be. Thus, sugar pills may reduce pain, and – as we will see in Chapter 6 – nearly half of all depressed patients improve on a placebo.

Less familiar is the possibility that drugs themselves, even if they are not inert, also have powerful placebo effects. Thus a patient may not respond to an antidepressant not because of a specific effect on the brain, but because of a powerful expectation that the drug will work.

Physicians are often puzzled when a drug works well for a few months, and then seems to become ineffective. Consider for example, the phenomenon of "antidepressant tolerance" (popularly called "Prozac poopout"). Patients initially do well on the drug, and then it just doesn't seem to work at all (Baldessarini, Ghaemi, and Viguera, 2002).

What is happening here? Is there some mysterious mechanism by which the brain goes back into "chemical imbalance?" A more likely explanation is that initial improvement on an antidepressant was a placebo effect that was mistaken for a therapeutic effect. Since such phenomena are difficult to study, it is not always clear that when drugs stop working, one is seeing "treatment resistance."

2.8 CLINICAL GUIDELINES

For most practitioners, following the psychopharmacology literature can be confusing. One reads so many claims – and so many contradictions. Rather than have to find one's own way through a research morass, it is advantageous to have guidelines written by experts.

The American Psychiatric Association (APA) publishes a series of clinical guidelines for the management of common mental disorders, offered as printed supplements to the *American Journal of Psychiatry*, and on the web. In the UK, the National Institute for Clinical Excellence (NICE) has published about 50 guidelines for psychiatric treatment.

Both sets of documents have come to be considered benchmarks. Guidelines written by experts are often seen as authoritative. Some psychiatrists even hesitate to practice outside of these recommendations, wondering how their treatment might stand up in court if things were to go wrong.

However clinical guidelines can be no better than the current state of research evidence. Which is to say, they cannot be scientific documents. Undoubtedly, expert consensus is usually better than individual clinical opinion. But experts are perfectly capable of getting things wrong. That is particularly likely when diseases are not well understood, and when RCTs are thin on the ground.

Moreover, guidelines are developed around the current diagnostic system – which is to say they are built on sand. How can one write guidelines for the treatment of major depression if this category is a heterogeneous group of conditions, each of which may require different treatment methods?

Another problem is that even when clinical guidelines are based on the best available evidence, the evidence may just not be good enough. You need to get past the authoritative tone of final documents and look at the actual studies that recommendations are based on. You may be in for a shock. Much has been based on very little.

Last but not least, experts have their own biases – theoretical positions to defend and axes to grind. Many of those who write clinical guidelines are deeply committed to aggressive pharmacotherapy, and have little interest in the alternatives. Moreover, most experts in psychopharmacology are receiving funding in one form or another from pharmaceutical companies (see Chapter 3). Even if experts do not believe they are being directly influenced by industry funding, it is likely to play a role in their views. That provides still another reason why published guidelines should not be taken as scripture.

In the end, the recommendations of any committee tend to be compromises between several strongly held (but far from proven) ideas about treatment. And where the data is unclear, conclusions will be influenced by the views of whoever has been chosen to be on the committee. The final conclusions are often political – a compromise between factions rather than a scientifically based conclusion. Moreover, guidelines have often been written to help clinicians manage situations for which there is little or no evidence about how to proceed.

In summary, while the science of drug therapy continues to advance, real-world practice is only partly evidence-based. Some of my colleagues are natural enthusiasts who want to give their patients the benefit of the latest (and most "aggressive") treatment. That usually means prescribing drugs off-label, without waiting for the results of clinical trials.

My view is just the opposite. The limitations of scientific evidence should make us more conservative and cautious in prescribing drugs. If psychiatry were based more firmly on science, practice would look quite different. Fewer drugs would be prescribed, and polypharmacy would be less common. Newer drugs would not be favored over older drugs that are just as effective. Alternatives to psychopharmacology would be more often considered. That is the message of this book.

CHAPTER 3

The Pharmaceutical Industry

Pharmaceutical development should ideally be driven by science and public health. But in practice, drug development is determined more by marketing than by research.

This is a problem that afflicts all of medicine – not just psychiatry. There has been some formal research about the influence of industry on the practice of medicine, and two substantive books have been published on the subject (Angell, 2005; Avorn, 2004). The data show that drug companies have an inordinate influence on prescribing practices. And much of that influence comes from the funding of academic physicians.

3.1 THE PHARMACEUTICAL INDUSTRY AND ACADEMIC PSYCHIATRY

Drug companies are corporations, driven by profit and risk. The pharmaceutical industry, sometimes called "Big Pharma" because of its size, is the most lucrative of *all* business enterprises. That was not true in the past. The transformation took place as indications for drugs expanded.

Patients who are medically ill have access to many effective drugs. But a much broader market has opened up among those who are well but seek to *avoid* illness (e.g., taking statins to lower cholesterol). There is also a wider market among those whose symptoms are

The Use and Misuse of Psychiatric Drugs: An Evidence-Based Critique   by Joel Paris
© 2010 John Wiley & Sons, Ltd

troubling but would not ordinarily require treatment (as in the therapy of milder forms of depression).

The treatment of common mental disorders (milder anxiety and depression) has been extremely lucrative for industry. This is a market that could, in principle, include a large percentage of the world's population. These are some of the developments that have made pharmaceuticals into a multi-billion dollar industry. And as the stakes for success become higher, companies have been spending more money on marketing than on research.

To protect its market share, Big Pharma uses some of its profits to obtain political influence. The pharmaceutical industry has enormous clout – on both sides of the Atlantic. But its power is particularly striking in the USA, a country ideologically committed to private enterprise and suspicious of government regulation. American political campaigns cost a good deal of money, a fact that opens the door for industry to make political contributions to influence Congressmen to act on their behalf. While one cannot show direct links, it is hard to believe that the passage of legislation allowing pharmaceutical companies in the USA to directly advertise to consumers had nothing to do with the large sums they provided to many Congressmen for re-election.

Money can also be used to bring the medical profession onside. Big Pharma uses a variety of strategies to accomplish that goal. Academic physicians are particularly important for industry because they are influential – or are, in the current jargon, "key opinion-leaders" (KOLs). Unlike scientists directly employed by companies, academics come with the prestige of great universities. Professors at medical schools are highly credible. They give talks at conventions, at hospitals, and at universities attended by many practitioners. Industry values the support of KOLs and is prepared to pay for it.

How do they do this? First, drug companies involve academics in clinical research on their products, directly sponsored by industry. In the past, governments supported some of these trials. Today, obtaining public funding for RCTs is much more difficult (and highly competitive). With a decline in peer-reviewed grants, clinical trials, always a high priority in academic medicine, are being supported almost entirely by pharmaceutical companies (Dove, 2000).

This situation has led to serious bias in research methods and reporting. To put the matter bluntly, industry is in a position to buy the scientific results it needs to market its products. It has been empirically shown that industry-sponsored trials are significantly more likely to support their products (Perlis *et al.*, 2005). As we will see, there are several ways of making sure that published results favor the company that paid for the trial. Over time, RCTs have become more expensive, and it is hard to imagine how governments could carry them out alone. But the domination of industry introduces a profit motive into what should be obejctive scientific research.

Why do academics get involved in this process? One reason is that clinical trials are an important source of funding for researchers. (Not necessarily for their personal use – money left over is often used for other projects.) Moreover, clinical research is crucially important for universities and hospitals, which take a percentage of the funds to support their activities. These benefits help to explain why there has been little regulation of clinical trial procedures. This is a good example of the principle that – as recent economic events have shown – the engine of capitalism, however much it drives wealth and progress, requires regulation.

To be fair, the researchers who run clinical trials, the administrators who support them, and the companies that fund them believe that new drugs can help patients. But the large amounts of money involved have a definite potential to corrupt.

Second, industry has significant influence on whether drugs will be approved. The reason is that the government agencies assigned to approve marketing of new drugs call on the services of the same academic physicians, who are in turn KOLs (Avorn, 2006). Since these experts receive part of their income from industry, for both ideological and practical reasons, they are sympathetic to the introduction of new drugs.

Third, industry directly funds academics to carry out tasks expected of KOLs. Psychiatric professors often give lectures that subtly (or unsubtly) favor pharmaceutical products (Healy and Thase, 2003). Universities, as well as granting agencies (such as the National Institute of Mental Health in the USA) recognize this potential conflict of interest, and require any income from this source to be reported. A common policy of universities is to take back any payments that exceed a ceiling. However, as we will see, the procedure has not been consistently enforced.

Fourth, industry can provide academic physicians who are KOLs with "consulting" fees (Avorn, 2004). Since the process of consultation is often pro forma, these fees are actually indirect payments for supporting a product. The amounts can sometimes be quite large, as will be seen in some of the examples to be discussed below.

Many academic psychiatrists make less money than they could if they were working outside a university. For this reason it is tempting to accept industry largesse. KOLs who publish clinical research are invited to go on tour to visit hospitals across their own country (or internationally), presenting their data – while staying at the best hotels and eating gourmet dinners. Some even use power point presentations prepared by the company (in which case the slide designs can be rather impressive). But even speakers who prepare their own talks are unlikely to present data that contradict the message of the sponsoring company.

Another temptation that industry provides to researchers is to make life easy by writing articles for them, to which they only need attach their name. The practice of ghostwriting has been of great concern to journal editors (Flanagin and Rennie, 1995). It raises serious questions about the scientific quality of what is published in scientific journals (Healy and Cattell, 2003).

Putting all these questionable practices together, it has become very difficult to find a professor of psychiatry whose opinion can be fully trusted to reflect science rather than the influence of industry. The question has been raised about academic medicine (Angell, 2000) – and about academic psychiatry in particular (Healy and Thase, 2003) – whether the profession is up for sale.

This is not to say that anyone who accepts money from industry must always be corrupted. However, there needs to be limits on these relationships. Government agencies should support more clinical trials. And KOLs should not be allowed to earn millions by supporting pharmaceutical products, even if these new drugs benefit patients. The role of academic physicians should be to weigh the evidence for and against any innovation, and to be conservative about drugs until they have been on the market for enough time to determine their real effectiveness. This means that the activities of KOLs have to be carefully regulated, under rules that are actually enforced. As we will see, that has not always been the case.

3.2 THE COUNTERATTACK ON CONFLICT OF INTEREST

The problem of keeping industry influence away from academic medicine has been highlighted, not only in medical journals, but also in the media, and in investigations by lawmakers. The most prominent critic has been an American Senator from Iowa, Charles Grassley, who has taken on conflicts of interest in academic medicine as a special cause. Although Grassley is a conservative Republican who came into the Senate during the presidency of Ronald Reagan (and who strongly opposes national health insurance), on this issue, almost every end of the political spectrum could consider him as a hero.

One of the main problems raised by Grassley is that professional medical organizations receive a large part of their funding from industry. For this reason, psychiatric associations cannot speak on behalf of the public interest without endangering their own financial structure. Grassley challenged the American Psychiatric Association (APA) to show why, given the fact that 30% of its budget comes from industry, its positions are not tainted (Moran, 2008). In a series of recommendations published by a group of journal editors and heads of professional medical associations (including the current CEO of the American Psychiatric Association), it was proposed, rather conservatively, that a cap of no more than 25% of total budget be based on such contributions.

These recommendations are now being put into practice by the APA, which is closing down the industry-sponsored symposia that have been a feature of its large annual meeting. In fact this decision has already led to the APA conference being one day shorter as of 2010, showing just how essential pharmaceutical money was for the organization. The World Psychiatric Association had already restricted industry funding for its meetings from 2009.

There are other indications that the problems described in this chapter are being corrected as a result of a backlash against the scope of industry influence on professional organizations. In several countries, including the UK, industry has agreed to abide by common rules concerning what their representatives can give to physicians.

Another problem for professional organizations is that they elect officers who can be senior professors in the pay of industry. Even if these physicians give up their perks while in office, if they may have made large profits in the past, they can no longer be considered unbiased. Rothman *et al.* (2009) suggested that leaders of these associations should be free of industry involvement for several *years* prior to taking up these roles.

Senator Grassley specifically asked whether the public should be concerned about whether the president of the APA for 2009–2010, Alan Schatzberg, Chair of Psychiatry at Stanford University, can be an independent voice for his profession. Schatzberg, a well-known researcher, was reported to have a $6 million stake in a company making a drug that he has been studying, with his wife having a $4.8 million investment in another drug development company (*New York Times*, July 12, 2008). While Schatzberg has denied that these involvements constitute a conflict of interest, the facts are troubling.

It would be illustrative to review some recent and prominent examples of how scenarios for conflict of interest have become apparent. Each case shows how Big Pharma can seriously corrupt the higher levels of academic psychiatry.

Conflict of interest in academic psychiatry arises when researchers are in a position to profit personally by promoting drugs, either through their published research, or by giving lectures and symposia. Even if they *think* they are objective, they cannot be under the circumstances.

One would like to believe that problems are exceptional, particularly at the higher levels of academic leadership. But in fact conflicts of interest are common among the most famous psychiatrists in North America.

Charles Nemeroff, one of the world's leading researchers in psychopharmacology, and for many years a department chair at Emory University in Atlanta, has had a series of problems of this nature (*New York Times*, June 8, 2008). The first occurred when Nemeroff wrote a paper published in *Nature Neuroscience* (Nemeroff and Owens, 2003) presenting evidence in favor of a transdermal patch to administer lithium. What Nemeroff did not reveal to the journal was that he held a patent for this device (and that he was a paid consultant to two dozen pharmaceutical and biotech companies). A protest letter was sent to the journal by two other researchers (Carroll and Rubin, 2003), insisting that standards for transparency about conflict of interest should be maintained by a journal as prestigious as *Nature*. In response, Nemeroff and Owens (2003) pointed out that they had not technically violated journal standards (since this was a review article). Nonetheless, the choice not to disclose raises questions.

In a second incident, Nemeroff was forced to resign as editor of the journal *Neuropsychopharmacology* in 2006 for failing to disclose financial conflicts of interest. This time he had published a paper (Nemeroff *et al.*, 2006) supporting a device made by Cyberonics Inc. for vagus nerve stimulation as a treatment for depression. But Nemeroff did not report the large payments he had received from Cyberonics.

In a third incident, Nemeroff was forced to resign as Chair of Psychiatry at Emory in 2008. Senator Grassley revealed that Nemeroff had received millions of dollars from industry, and failed to report this income, as required by university and NIMH regulations. Although he is one of the leading and most respected psychiatrists in the USA, once he was shown to have broken the rules, Nemeroff had to pay the price.

If a psychiatrist as prominent as Nemeroff could fall from grace due to conflict of interest, how many others are involved? We do not know for sure, but there have been several other cases. The National Institutes of Mental Health (NIMH), which is supposed to be an independent government agency supporting high quality research, became concerned that some of its researchers were receiving millions from pharmaceutical companies. In 2005, it introduced a policy in which its employees can no longer receive *any* income from industry. And academics receiving grants from NIMH were also required to report any conflicts of interest. As the *New York Times* (June 8, 2008) described, the policy was: "to protect research integrity, the National Institutes of Health require researchers to report to universities earnings of $10,000 or more per year, for instance, in consulting money from makers of drugs also studied by the researchers in federally financed trials."

Most universities have similar regulations, requiring that all payments from industry be disclosed. But these rules are more honored in the breach than in the observance. *The New York Times* (June 8, 2008) reported that Martin Keller, Chair of Psychiatry at Brown University, and a leading researcher on antidepressants, had earned more than a million dollars from companies whose drugs he supported (through articles in medical journals as well as conference presentations). This conflict of interest must have been well known (working at another university, I heard people talking about it for years), yet action was only taken when the matter was publicized in a newspaper.

A similar problem afflicted Joseph Biederman, a well-known child psychiatrist at the Massachusetts General Hospital and Harvard University. The *New York Times* article (June 8, 2008) reported that Biederman, along with two other Harvard professors, belatedly reported $1.6 million in income from the pharmaceutical industry. A prominent researcher on attention-deficit hyperactivity disorder (ADHD), Biederman has widely promoted the use of drugs to treat children with behavioral disturbances. He is also one of the most prominent supporters of the use of mood stabilizers and neuroleptics for what he and his supporters consider to be childhood bipolar disorder (see Chapter 7).

Fred Goodwin, a well-known American psychiatrist and a former director of NIMH, ran into a similar problem. Goodwin has conducted important research on bipolar disorders, and is the co-author of a major textbook on the subject (Goodwin and Jamison, 2007). But Senator Grassley discovered that Goodwin had a conflict of interest, in that he took payments for travel and drug talks from industry, totaling $2.8 million over seven years (*New York Times*, November 22, 2008).

Goodwin had long hosted a program on National Public Radio, "The Infinite Mind," which described new developments in psychiatry for the educated public. In his role as journalist, Goodwin had agreed to report any conflicts due to payments for lectures from drug companies. He did not do so. Since these fees contravened the policy of the radio network, Goodwin's participation in the show was terminated.

Interestingly, Goodwin stated that it had never occurred to him that there was any problem, as taking industry money for lectures was a normal procedure in academic medicine. With respect to the culture of medical academia, Goodwin was absolutely correct. Taking money from industry has been so much a part of the landscape that very few people notice it.

No doubt most of the physicians who accept these fees are convinced that nothing they say was *directly* influenced by industry. But anyone who believes that professional opinions are in no way influenced by financial support has to be naïve. It is not a question of company representatives whispering in their ears, but of a shared belief in the unique value of drugs that are being actively promoted by industry. Consciously or not, what one says (and believes) is influenced by who pays the bill.

All these examples suggest that the opinions expressed by academic experts, as well as the clinical guidelines based on these opinions, cannot necessarily be trusted. It is now clear that problems with financial gain involve some of the most prominent and influential psychiatrists in the US, who have had the power to influence how drugs are prescribed. There are hardly any KOLs in the field of psychopharmacology who have not financially benefited from industry support. And billions of dollars in sales are affected by what they have to say.

Even if this issue has only now exploded in the media, it is most certainly not new. Earlier concerns about conflict of interest led to the development of requirements for transparency. Researchers giving talks must list the companies that have paid them whenever they speak or publish an article. For some, the list is long. Some believe that if they take money from almost every company, that proves their neutrality (Lexchin *et al.*, 2003). But that conclusion is contradicted by the fact that research funded by industry consistently tends to produce results that support the products under study.

It can be argued that clinical trials will always depend to some extent on industry, that governments will always be tight-fisted, and that some research cannot be carried out in any other way. But even if that were so, academic psychiatrists do not need to make *millions* from drug companies. They already earn a comfortable income from universities, hospitals, and clinical practice.

The tragedy is that academic medicine is losing the luster it gained over many decades by its leadership in advancing medical treatment. Instead of being role models, that is, putting science and the public interest ahead of personal gain, too many leading academics have been models of the greed and poor judgment that have created a crisis for the world as a whole.

3.3   THREATS TO THE INTEGRITY OF CLINICAL TRIALS

The bottom-line message for psychiatrists is that the results of clinical trials conducted by industry cannot be trusted. How does Big Pharma pull the wool over our eyes? When all clinical trials are paid by and conducted under their supervision, they not only foot the bill, but set up the protocols and analyze the data. That is the reason why results are so much more likely to come out the way the company wants (Lexchin *et al.*, 2003; Perlis *et al.*, 2005; Heres *et al.*, 2006).

Moreover, if findings do not support the product under study, the results may not be published. The suppression of negative findings in an industry-sponsored clinical trial unfolded into a scandal a few years ago in Canada (Olivieri, 2003). A prominent hematologist, Nancy Olivieri, stopped tests of a new drug (deferiprone) for thalassemia because she concluded from preliminary data that the agent could be dangerous. However, when she attempted to inform the public about these problems, the company sued her for breaking a contract she had signed promising secrecy. Olivieri even lost her job for a time, although the President of the University of Toronto eventually reinstated her. In this example, industry was willing to destroy a researcher's career because she put their profits from drug development at risk.

It has now come to wide attention how often suppression of less than positive (or negative) results can occur. Researchers now have access to the results of both published and unpublished data. For antidepressants, when the results of unpublished trials are included in a meta-analysis, evidence for efficacy becomes much weaker (Turner *et al.*, 2008; Kirsch *et al.*, 2008).

That is one of the reasons why a new system of reporting has now been instituted. Clinical trials must be registered with government agencies, to ensure that negative results cannot be hidden (DeAngelis *et al.*, 2004).

Yet even without actively suppressing data, industry can manipulate results in a positive direction. The easiest is to choose patient samples using inclusion and exclusion criteria that make a good outcome more likely. As discussed in Chapter 2, people who sign up for trials are a special group (less sick and more compliant than patients physicians see in practice). If patients are not allowed to be "comorbid" for other mental disorders, they may be more likely to improve, even if clinical reality presents us with a majority of cases that are comorbid, complex, and much more resistant to treatment. Again, trials rarely compare new drugs to existing agents, but load the dice by making placebo comparisons only, which avoid reaching the conclusion that a new and expensive drug is no better than older and cheaper alternatives already on the market. Another trick that has sometimes been used is to publish secondary analyses, suggesting that sub-groups of patients might have benefited, even when the sample as a whole did not. All these problems compromise the clinical relevance of results from drug trials.

Once a drug is shown to be effective in a clinical trial, it has to be government approved in order to be marketed. In the US, when clinical trials are successful, new drugs are submitted to the Food and Drug Administration (FDA) for approval. In the UK, the Medicines and Healthcare Products Regulatory Agency (MHRA) makes these decisions.

Unfortunately, the bar for putting a new agent on the market is not very high. It only takes a few clinical trials that point in the right direction. Many of these trials are paid for by the manufacturer. This places doubt on their validity. Moreover, the regulators who make these decisions are themselves in conflict interest, since most have received industry funding.

To get a product on the market rapidly, industry can work to influence government agencies directly. It is not generally known that the FDA itself, as well as the MHRA, are funded with industry money. And most experts asked to participate in decisions have been on an industry payroll. Up to recently, no members of FDA panels had to rescue themselves if they were receiving money from the companies whose products they were assessing. A new set of guidelines has only recently been instituted to correct the problem.

Actually, since nearly every leading psychopharmacologist has close ties to industry, it is almost impossible to find an expert who is *not* receiving substantial fees from drug companies. This conundrum shows how deeply medical science has been compromised by financial gain. The culture has to be changed with regulations to prevent researchers from profiting from their own findings. If there were rules of this kind – and if they were enforced – most academics would choose to protect their reputations rather than put them at risk.

With all these problems in mind, you need to carefully read published clinical trials to see who paid for them. If pharmaceutical funding was involved, they should not be taken at face value. I teach my students to doubt the validity of any journal article in which a trial had industry support.

If our society wants better drugs, it needs to invest in research. In the past, the National Institute of Mental Health paid for drug trials, and also supported research in which drugs were compared to non-pharmacological forms of treatment (e.g., Elkin *et al.*, 1989) – something industry *never* does. Public funding is necessary to restore confidence in the integrity of clinical trials.

3.4 THE LIMITS OF INDUSTRY POWER

When an industry is as large and as powerful as major pharmaceutical companies, it must inevitably exert a major influence on academic psychiatry. Yet some have ascribed even more power to Big Pharma than it actually holds. For a fictional example of this "paranoid" view, read the best-selling thriller "The Constant Gardener" (LeCarré, 2001).

It is sometimes imagined that companies lurk behind the scenes to manipulate decisions made by academics, and that they control the university by threatening withdrawal of financial support if anyone fails to toe their line. By and large, that is *not* how things work. Pharmaceutical companies prefer to exert their influence in more subtle ways. Since university departments of psychiatry depend on their support, pharmaceutical companies do not need to make explicit and heavy-handed threats. They prefer to create bonds with academics that are seen as partnerships promoting mutual interests. And most professors of psychiatry are comfortable seeing themselves as partners, not servants of industry.

In 2000, an incident in Canada stirred up a storm of worldwide interest in the media about the extent of industry influence on a department of psychiatry (Healy, 2004). David Healy, a well-known psychopharmacological researcher from the University of Cardiff, was offered a professorship at the University of Toronto. Healy, who has contributed greatly to our understanding of psychopharmacology and its limitations (Healy, 2002, 2009), holds some controversial views on the relationship between SSRIs and the risk of suicide. The trouble in Toronto occurred when, in a lecture given while he was visiting the university, Healy stated that SSRI antidepressants can be dangerous, and might even be responsible for thousands of excess deaths through completed suicide.

That relationship is still being debated (see Chapter 6), and at this point most experts (e.g., Cipriani, Barbul, and Geddes, 2005) have concluded that SSRIs can increase suicidal thoughts and behaviors, but do not lead to completed suicide. However senior academics in Toronto were alarmed by Healy's views, presented publicly and with strong rhetoric. They did not want a leader who questioned the medical and ethical value of prescribing the drugs they gave patients every day. Toronto rescinded its job offer, a decision made within days of the lecture.

One could argue whether or not the right decision was made, or whether the process was fair. But a good story always tends to trump the muddled truth of events. The sequence of events led to suspicion that the pharmaceutical industry had intervened behind the scenes to force the university to silence Healy. Eli Lilly, the company that manufactures Prozac, had recently given a multi-million dollar gift to the University of Toronto. (The donation was not directly connected to drug trials, but funded a renovated floor for medical education.) If you read anything about the incident today, particularly on the web, the idea that Lilly was responsible for Healy losing his job offer is the one that predominates. Actually there is no evidence that Lilly was involved in withdrawing the job offer. But the idea became a received wisdom, in part supported by Healy himself – both on the internet and in published books (Healy, 2004).

The other issue raised by the Healy story was academic freedom. Professors are supposed to be free to express unpopular views. The Canadian Association of University Teachers protested the incident, viewing it as a breach of these principles. However, when it comes to issues that affect public health, academic freedom cannot be considered absolute.

In my view, Healy had a legitimate grievance about the hiring process, since he had made definite plans to move from Cardiff to Toronto. He was eventually, and rightly, compensated by a financial settlement.

Yet academic freedom is not really under threat. In the end, KOLs are in no way forced to support the aims of industry. They can simply decide to be honest – and reduce their income. There have always been – and still are – severe critics of Big Pharma in medical schools. But academics who opposed their goals, such as the American psychiatrist Leon Eisenberg (2000), did not conduct clinical trials. The people who take industry money to do research have more reason to be careful about criticism. That is where conflicts of interest are most likely.

In summary, the problem is not a John LeCarré-like conspiracy, but an implicit understanding that academics who take money from industry will support its products. In this way, the question, "is academic psychiatry for sale?", is not just rhetorical.

The picture I have drawn of the pharmaceutical industry is not a pretty one. To be fair, drug companies have also done much good for the public, and many of us (including myself) depend on their products to stay healthy. But when the industry became a behemoth, its power got out of hand.

We should not expect pharmaceutical executives, who are responsible to their stockholders, to search after scientific truth. Nor should we blame the industry for promoting its products. It is up to us to live up to a higher standard. If there is a problem, academic psychiatrists have no one else but themselves to blame.

3.5 INDUSTRY AND THE PRACTICING PSYCHIATRIST

Industry can also influence physician behavior in ways that do not involve academic opinion leaders. They can make direct contact with practitioners. Fees can be paid, directly or indirectly, to high-prescribing doctors who are influential in their medical communities. Industry may invite these physicians to attend meetings at expensive resorts – again calling the process a "consultation." In some cases, the companies actually pay physicians for every prescription they write (Avorn, 2006). The means are often deceptive, and some practitioners have been personally reimbursed for enrolling patients in clinical trials.

The pharmaceutical industry not only supports the professional associations to which most psychiatrists belong, but members can sometimes attend scientific meetings for free, if drug representatives pay for air fare and hotel. (This practice, while not universal, is all too common.)

The most direct way of marketing a product is to advertise it. Pharmaceutical ads appear in medical journals. They claim to provide information, but are basically little but well-presented deceptions. A normal part of any business is advertising. And when you are promoting a product, you put things in the best possible light. Advertisements in medical journals are glossy, expensive, and highly effective (Angell, 2004). For this reason, some have questioned whether drug promotions should be allowed in scientific publications. There have even been cases in which industry has punished journals for critical comments about their products by removing advertising (Lexchin and Light, 2006).

On the other hand, without advertisements, medical journals (including the one that I currently edit) would have to close down. Someone has to pay the bill. But as more and more journals go on line, advertising might become less central to their operations.

The actual content of drug advertising is not very informative. One often sees a large photo of an attractive young woman (even when the drug in question is usually prescribed for people who are not necessarily attractive). While all possible side effects of a drug must be acknowledged in these ads, they are listed in very small print.

Needless to say, claims of efficacy for drugs in these advertisements are never vetted. One must assume that industry *always* distorts the evidence. Positive studies will be presented out of context, with no balance between good and bad results (up to recently, negative findings were entirely suppressed). The ads focus on selective studies financed by industry itself (but authored by KOLs).

Moreover, drugs are only advertised when they are new, that is, when the data on them is still slim. Older drugs, even when still under patent, may not be promoted. While more is known about these agents, they are not "the latest thing."

Yet drug advertisements are not the main way for industry to get its message out to physicians. Much more important is the use of pharmaceutical representatives (Elliott, 2003). Selling drugs to doctors requires a personal touch. Pharmaceutical representatives or "detail men" (now more often women) go out to physician's offices and convince doctors to try new drugs. Drug reps are salespeople, chosen for their interpersonal skills (they are uniformly charming and engaging). Drug reps establish a personal contact, presenting themselves as enablers for a physician's work. They knock on doors, give out pamphlets, and ask for time to talk about their product.

Many physicians want to give new drugs a try. Hands-on experience makes them comfortable. They do not consider that placebo effects can be stronger for a new drug than an old one. When the agent is novel, enthusiasm and curiosity make it seem to work better. (It is an old saying in medicine, sometimes attributed to William Osler, that physicians should hasten to use new drugs before they stop working.)

Thus, the latest drugs tend to sell because they are new, and not because they are better. In internal medicine, a large-scale study (The ALLHAT Collaborative Research Group, 2002) showed that classical diuretics, which are generic and cheap, are more effective for hypertension than any newer alternatives (ACE inhibitors or calcium channel blockers), most of which are on patent and expensive. But medical practice did not change at all as a result of this finding. Prescribing a "golden oldie" like chlorthiazide was not very appealing. Similarly, Gaziano, Opie, and Weinstein (2006) found that acetyl salicylic acid, plus one of the older anti-hypertensives, could provide effective reduction of most cardiovascular diseases – a cheap alternative for developing countries. But in most places practice remained dependent on the newest drugs.

Finally, marketing requires monitoring. In some communities industry has access to data showing who is (and who is not) prescribing their product (Avorn, 2006). This information allows them to reward physicians who do what they want, and to recruit those not yet onside by visiting them in their offices (and by providing gifts).

Drug companies often respond to criticism of their high profits by pointing out that they invest heavily in research. If only that were true! Drug companies spend most of their budgets on marketing. The reality is that only a small percentage of industry profits go into drug development (Angell, 2005). We badly need new and innovative drugs, but developing them involves significant financial risk. That is why most new agents are "me-too" drugs that differ little from those already on the market. Industry does conduct research, but there is more profit in selling drugs than in creating them.

To be fair, Big Pharma provides unrestricted grants for medical education. When I was in charge of meetings and rounds at my hospital, I was grateful for this kind of support. But that is a pittance compared to the salaries industry pays for an army of pharmaceutical representatives.

For drug advertisements, and for visits from "drug reps," nothing forces us to take anything they say seriously. Physicians should always be skeptical about claims for new drugs. To practice evidence-based medicine, we need to read journals critically and ignore disinformation. We also need to avoid relying on industry for information. Finally, we should also be skeptical about sponsored talks and conferences by KOLs. Unfortunately, busy practitioners do not always feel ready to investigate these matters on their own. That is why disseminating information through biased sources is so effective for industry.

Industry knows that all its strategies for obtaining the support of psychiatrists are highly successful. Most physicians accept what industry tells them. To demonstrate the influence of marketing, one need only note that the moment a drug goes generic, the frequency of its prescription goes down almost immediately (Avorn, 2006). That is because pharmaceutical representatives stop marketing them.

Actually, industry has a few tricks up its sleeve when products go generic. They can introduce a metabolite of the original drug – a strategy often used to market a competitive agent (e.g., pregabalin instead of gabapentin). Another popular ploy has been to introduce an extended release form of the original, as has happened for venlafalxine, quetiapine, and methylphenidate. This strategy fools physicians into believing that the new product is preferable. Actually almost all psychiatric drugs can be given once daily – the metabolism of drugs provides an "extended release" of its own).

3.6   GIFTS TO PHYSICIANS

Research convincingly demonstrates that giving gifts to physicians influences their prescribing practices (Wazana, 2000; Campbell *et al.*, 2007). Physicians themselves may think that accepting gifts does not change their choices in any way. But the data clearly show that such investments pay off, making physicians significantly more likely to prescribe industry products.

Each year the American Psychiatric Association holds a large convention, attracting as many as 20,000 practitioners, from both the USA and the rest of the world. One of the most striking features of this event has been the exhibit hall, where each pharmaceutical company has had a booth. In addition to information about products, each company offers attendees gifts of some kind. The items can vary from pens to calculators. None are particularly expensive – and one might ask why reasonably well-paid psychiatrists need such things for free. But there is something irresistible about a "freebie." One sees colleagues coming out of the hall with "loot bags" filled with these presents. It may seem unimportant if a physician uses a Prozac pen (as opposed to a pen advertising some other product). But whether one admits it or not, one is more likely to prescribe Prozac when one sees the name every day. (Recently, industry has agreed to stop giving out pens, but has not changed many of its other practices.)

Food can also be used as a gift. For many years, at the APA conference, you could go to breakfast meetings every morning and attend dinner meetings every evening. (The only thing missing was a free lunch.) It was only under the pressure of bad publicity that a decision to discontinue industry-sponsored symposia at APA meetings was made.

Drug companies also sponsor talks by academic luminaries who come to various cities when they are "on the circuit." Typically these events are held in some of the best restaurants in town, places where most physicians would only go on a special occasion. But there is no bill to pay – industry covers all the costs.

Many companies have accepted regulations against giving more expensive gifts. In fact, most industry guidelines preclude paying for hotels and travel. But many companies do it anyway. And as noted, psychiatrists can sometimes be invited to travel to exotic locations as part of a consulting fee, even though they are not being consulted about anything in particular. And some practitioners have received payment just to attend conferences. Industry is not interested in their opinion, but in shaping their prescribing.

Pharmaceutical representatives work to cultivate relationships with physicians early in their careers, when they are still students or residents (Hodges, 1995). They have been known to buy stethoscopes for poor (or not so poor) medical students. In psychiatry, they sponsor parties for residents, or pay for pizza to encourage attendance at Journal Clubs. (Some universities have begun to ban this practice.)

By investing in trainees, industry hopes to establish lifetime loyalty among physicians. So the problem is not that trainees are corrupted by free lunches, but that a climate is created in which physicians are less likely to be cautious about accepting industry's views about drugs.

3.7   DIRECT ADVERTISING TO THE PUBLIC

The worst abuse of Big Pharma consists of direct advertising of their products to potential patients. This practice is currently allowed *only* in the USA and New Zealand. Years ago, no one would have imagined that pharmaceutical companies would ever be allowed to advertise their products directly to consumers. It was assumed that physicians, who are knowledgeable about drugs, are the ones who should make these decisions, and that patients are not in a position to judge the value of the prescribed agents.

Today we live in a more democratic age, when consumers are more involved in the choice of medical treatment. (Patients may walk into our offices with reprints downloaded from the internet.) Even so, most countries in the world continue to bar direct to consumer advertising.

The story behind this marketing practice is not pretty. Industry got the US Congress to change its laws about advertising to consumers in the same way as other powerful lobbies. Politicians always need money, and Big Pharma has no lack of funds. Buying Congressmen was a very smart investment on the part of industry.

Direct advertising has had a profound impact on how the public uses drugs. It has affected all pharmaceutical agents on the market.

(Viagra may be the most obvious example, but is far from the only one).

Although I live in Canada, where this practice is not formally allowed, we all see drug ads in American magazines or on American TV. One glossy advertisement in the *New York Times Magazine* was designed to convince people with mood problems that they are "really bipolar," suggestion that readers go to a web site called "isitjustdepression.com." Of course, that web site promotes just the kind of drug (a mood stabilizer) the company makes. A television ad, also directed at people who might have bipolar disorder, showed a beautiful young woman on the seashore (evidently fully recovered from her illness), and advised people to consider taking apripazole, (an atypical neuroleptic) if their antidepressant hasn't worked. Needless to say, there was no mention of the many other (and more evidence-based) alternatives. One can only laugh at the claim of industry that the purpose of direct advertising is to provide useful information to consumers. As a practitioner, I find these advertisements horrifying.

But direct to consumer advertising works. It has been shown to lead to increased prescription of specific drugs. A recent survey found that one in five Americans was prompted to call or visit their doctor to discuss an advertised drug (Mintzes *et al.*, 2002). Moreover, these requests were usually complied with (in spite of doctors' reservations about the appropriateness of the treatment). Needless to say, all magazine and television advertisements include the tag line "discuss this with your doctor." But not every physician is able or willing to resist requests of patients for advertised drugs. The response, assuming that clinical results with other options have not been dramatic, is likely to be "OK, let's try it."

3.8 INDUSTRY AND PSYCHIATRIC DIAGNOSIS

The categorization of mental disorders in the DSM system can only be described as highly inclusive (over 400 diagnoses are listed in the current manual). With each new edition, one sees more (not less) pages and more (not less) disorders. Illnesses may also be diagnosed in people who are having normal reactions to life events (Horwitz and Wakefield, 2007). These diagnostic concepts have led to greatly increased prescriptions of drugs – particularly mood stabilizers and atypical neuroleptics (Patten and Paris, 2008). Relatively new diagnoses, such as social phobia, have been promoted heavily by industry with the aim of putting millions of people on drug treatment (Wakefield *et al.*, 2004).

We lack a gold standard to determine what is and what isn't a mental disorder. Psychiatrists tend to favor a broad definition. In the US, where services are only partially insured, there may be some who want more patients. Other specialists may feel more important if almost everyone is in need of their services.

The drug companies lean the same way, but for a different reason. They need to find more customers. From the point of view of the pharmaceutical industry, the more people take drugs regularly, the better. For them, the ideal agent would be one used by everyone – whether normal or ill.

Thus, while the actual contents of the DSM manual do not reflect a direct influence by industry, pharmaceutical companies and psychiatrists share a mind-set. They both believe that almost everyone who has a psychological problem should be prescribed drugs.

This trend towards universal pharmacy has been inadvertently reinforced by epidemiological research. A very large number of people meet criteria for a psychiatric diagnosis, at least as defined by DSM-IV-TR (American Psychiatric Association, 2000). The large-scale National Comorbidity Study (Kessler *et al.*, 2005a) found a lifetime prevalence of over 50% for any DSM-defined disorder. Actually these numbers reflect the fact that DSM lists many less severe conditions for which people do not necessarily seek help. But such findings give the impression that mental disorders are ubiquitous. Even though these surveys used sophisticated epidemiology, their results depend entirely on the assumption that the current diagnostic categories are valid and meaningful.

Depression screening programs are also based on DSM criteria. The problem is that they tend to identify mild cases in the community, which, as we will see, may not need treatment, and do not usually respond to pharmacotherapy (Patten, 2008). This is how distress of all kinds can be "medicalized" (see Chapter 10).

The idea that a large percentage of the population meets criteria for a psychiatric diagnosis is associated with the recent trend to identify mental disorders early in life, even before they start. And as we will see in Chapter 8, prescriptions of drugs to children and adolescents have greatly increased. These potential patients may or may not be ill, but are thought to be at risk for developing an illness later in life.

All these trends are greatly in the interest of the pharmaceutical industry. If everyone who is sad or socially anxious takes an antidepressant, there are very large profits to be made. One therefore has to be concerned as to whether the DSM manual itself could be influenced, however indirectly, by industry priorities.

To its credit, the American Psychiatric Association has taken action to prevent that from happening. The members of the various committees for DSM-V (expected in 2012) are all expected to have minimal or no ties to industry, that is, a maximum of $10,000 in income from these sources. Because so many academics earn much more than that in industry fees, the process of vetting everyone on the various committees put back the DSM revision process a full year. One can only assume that this rule will be enforced more strictly than similar restrictions previously set by granting agencies and universities.

3.9   THE PRICE FOR INDUSTRY SUPPORT

My own view of the pharmaceutical industry has changed. For many years, I thought I could simply ignore what it was doing. After all, nobody ever forced me to write a prescription for any particular drug. Moreover, my own practice has always been conservative. I am rarely interested in using the latest drugs. My policy has always been to avoid prescribing any agent until it has been on the market for a few years, waiting until its side effects become better known. But even if I stand fast, most of my colleagues go with the flow, and give patients the latest drugs promoted by industry.

When I became a university department chair, I had a benign view of industry influence. (I live in Canada, where we don't often see the kind of money that American psychiatrists can make.) Big Pharma had, after all, developed some excellent products. I thought that academia and industry should cooperate towards a common goal. And my department depended on their funding to run conferences that brought in eminent experts from far away. (Universities never have money for that sort of thing.) Moreover, some productive faculty members were using industry money to conduct necessary clinical trials, and used the left-over funds to support other good research.

But I eventually learned that there is no such thing as a free lunch. The price psychiatry pays for industry support is too high. To protect patient care, the process of drug development and promotion badly needs regulation.

A first step has already been put into place, with the introduction of a clinical trials registry in the US. Access to this information has already allowed researchers to analyze unpublished data and come to more sober conclusions about the efficacy of drugs. But psychiatrists, universities, and governments need to do much more.

I recommend three simple measures: (1) adopt regulations to prevent industry from paying more than minimal fees to researchers; (2) adopt regulations to prevent industry from giving gifts to physicians; (3) adopt a ban on direct advertising to the public. Establishing and enforcing these rules would not prevent the pharmaceutical industry from making a reasonable profit. But the public would be better protected.

The constant pressure of industry for prescription of new drugs (particularly those still protected by patent) has negative consequences for patients. The most obvious problem is cost. Newer drugs are always much more expensive. Prescriptions for new drugs tend to overwhelm those for older drugs, especially those that are out of patent (Avorn, 2004). But many older drugs are often just as good, if not better. And newer drugs are less likely to have side effects that have not yet been identified. (It took a decade for us to realize that atypical neuroleptics can cause metabolic syndrome.)

A second price is that industry pressure leads to polypharmacy, the practice of prescribing multiple drugs to one patient. From the point of view of industry, this can only be a good thing. But from the point of view of patients, the more drugs they take, the more side effects they must endure.

A third price is that non-pharmacological methods of treatment are not generally available, even when they are more efficacious than most drugs on the market. While billions of dollars have been made on antidepressants that do not always work, there is hardly any money to send unhappy and troubled people to psychotherapists, the efficacy of whose methods are as well-proven as that of any drug for depression (see Chapter 12).

Up to now, regulation of industry's relationship to medicine has not been in any way strict or effective. In the April 1, 2009 issue of *JAMA*, a group of editors across the USA published recommendations for a new set of guidelines to regulate the relationship between professional medical associations, academic medicine, and the pharmaceutical industry (Rothman *et al.*, 2009). The suggested changes would be as follows:

(1) A complete ban on industry funding of annual meetings, and an overall cap on industry funding for professional organizations.
(2) Meetings would no longer include satellite symposia funded by industry.
(3) No gifts would be allowed for attendees at meetings.
(4) All research grants from industry would be peer-reviewed.
(5) Committees that write practice guidelines would be entirely free of industry influence.
(6) No professional publications would be sponsored by industry (although advertising would be allowed).
(7) Professional bodies must never endorse industry products.

The pharmaceutical industry has brought great benefits to humanity. Yet as historians know, great victories often lead to hubris and defeat. As modestly sized companies with good profits turned into Big Pharma, a pattern of corruption set in. Physicians, particularly academic physicians, failed take a stand for rational therapy over market-driven fads. Doing so might mean making less money. But most of us did not go into this line of work to become fabulously rich. Our sacred trust remains the health of our patients.

PART II

Drugs in Practice

CHAPTER 4

Antipsychotics: For Better or For Worse

Antipsychotics are often called *neuroleptics*. That is because of their calming effect on "nerves." But these drugs have specific effects on psychotic symptoms, and all clinical guidelines agree that they are necessary for the treatment for schizophrenia (American Psychiatric Association, 2004; NICE, 2009).

In an emergency, acute episodes of psychosis can sometimes be "brought down" in hours. And there is no substitute for antipsychotics in the maintenance therapy of schizophrenia, where compliance with long-term treatment significantly reduces the frequency of relapse (Thieda, Beard, and Richter, 2003). Finally, as will be discussed later, antipsychotics can be invaluable in mania and psychotic depression.

These drugs are one of the greatest triumphs of psychiatry, but they have their limitations. Antipsychotics do not cure schizophrenia. "Positive symptoms," such as hallucinations and delusions respond well, but "negative symptoms" involving social withdrawal, such as "flattening" of emotion, and loss of will and motivation, do not, and illogical thought patterns respond only moderately (Tamminga and Davis, 2007; Healy, 2009). We are still waiting for the day when research produces drugs that treat the *disease* of schizophrenia – not just its symptoms. It is also possible that schizophrenia, which must still be considered a syndrome, may eventually be divided into more than one disease – each requiring a different treatment.

Moreover, the now widespread use of antipsychotic drugs in non-psychotic patients is a dubious and "off-label" indication. Most of

The Use and Misuse of Psychiatric Drugs: An Evidence-Based Critique   by Joel Paris
© 2010 John Wiley & Sons, Ltd

these agents are profoundly sedating, which is why they are being widely prescribed for insomnia or agitation. However common in everyday practice, this indication has not been systematically researched – or sanctioned by official regulatory bodies. Although off-label uses are not always mistaken, we should be particularly careful with powerful drugs like these. Antipsychotics should be used only for patients who absolutely need them. Where possible, equally effective and less toxic alternatives should be preferred.

4.1 FIRST GENERATION ANTIPSYCHOTICS

The first-generation antipsychotics (*FGAs or typicals*) were breakthrough drugs, and are still effective, albeit rarely prescribed. The first group to be introduced were *phenothiazines*, particularly agents in the *aliphatic* sub-class. Chlorpromazine (CPZ), introduced in North America in 1954, was a standard drug for many years. However CPZ has many problems (Leucht *et al.*, 2003). This is a highly sedating drug that can rapidly bring acutely ill patients under control. But it has low potency – milligram for milligram, antipsychotic effects are not as strong as for high potency agents. Thus therapeutic effects require very large doses, associated with a danger of hypotension.

In out-patient management, chlorpromazine is also less than ideal, since its sedative side effects made many patients complain of feeling "drugged." These effects were sometimes therapeutically useful for patients who were agitated or highly insomniac. But when it comes to maintenance, particularly in a chronically psychotic population, tolerability is crucial for compliance.

Although few phenothiazines are as sedating as CPZ, all have troubling side effects. The most common is an extrapyramidal syndrome (EPS), marked by restlessness, abnormal movements, and lack of facial expression. Although antiParkinsonian drugs reduce these symptoms, they are difficult to eliminate completely.

Phenothiazines also have less common side effects that can affect almost every organ system in the body. The most worrying is neuroleptic malignant syndrome (NMS), which presents with rigidity, fever, autonomic instability and delirium (Caroff and Mann, 1993). Although rare, that syndrome is potentially fatal.

The second group of phenothiazines were *piperidines*, and the most commonly used drug was thioridazine. While an effective antipsychotic, this agent is associated with dangerous cardiotoxicity, as well as retinopathy (Fenton *et al.*, 2007). For this reason, thioridazine is now prescribed only occasionally, and in some countries it has been taken off the market.

The third group of phenothiazines were *piperazines*. This group has the most advantages, and should retain a place in clinical practice. Their side effect profile is much less worrying than with aliphatics or piperidines. While piperazines do not always have a high enough potency for the effective treatment of acute psychosis, they are very useful for maintenance. Many patients can be sustained on small doses that do not necessarily produce EPS. As will be discussed later in the chapter, piperazines have been shown to perform just as well as modern antipsychotics in the management of schizophrenia.

The most commonly used piperazines are trifluoperazine and perphenazine. Another drug in this group, fluphenazine, was the first FGA to be available in a long-term injectable form (as a decanoate), and was, for many years, a standard way of managing non-compliant patients with schizophrenia.

It is a safe bet that few young psychiatrists have had much experience with phenothiazines. But there is a second drug class among the classical antipsychotics called *butyrophenones*. Haloperidol was the first agent to be introduced. Because haloperidol is highly potent in small doses, it has been (and continues to be) a valuable tool in the emergency room (Joy, Adams, and Lawrie, 2006). On the other hand, haloperidol is not a good oral maintenance drug, mainly because of a high incidence of EPS (Schillevoort *et al.*, 2001).

Even so, haloperidol worked. For years it was the gold standard of antipsychotic treatment, and was widely used in its decanoate form as a long-term injectable. It lost popularity because too many patients developed neurological side effects. These problems might have been avoided if patients who had been treated acutely with haloperidol had been switched to a piperazine after being discharged from hospital. All too often, whatever drug is prescribed in the emergency room tends to be continued for years to come. One wonders if FGAs as a group have been seen in an unfair light because of the wide use of haldoperidol as a maintenance drug in the 1970s and 1980s.

There is one crucial side effect that has made FGAs unpopular for the maintenance treatment of schizophrenia. The long-term use of phenothiazines and butyrophenones is associated with the development of tardive dyskinesia. That syndrome, characterized by abnormal movements of the tongue and the extremities, can emerge after patients take antipsychotics for several years (Gupta *et al.*, 2004). Tardive dyskinesia, unlike EPS, tends to get worse over time, and while it may remit when neuroleptics are removed at an early stage, once a severe case develops, no other drug is known to reverse it. While EPS can usually be managed with antiParkinsonian agents, there is no good way to manage tardive dyskinesia.

Tardive dyskinesia is most frequent with high-dose therapy of high potency agents, and its incidence in prospective studies has been as high as 5% a year (Correl *et al.*, 2004). It is even more likely to develop in elderly patients. In a prospective study of patients over age 55 given antipsychotic treatment (Woerner *et al.*, 1998), the cumulative rates after one, two and three years of tardive dyskinesia were 25, 34, and 53%.

One can easily see why concern about tardive dyskinesia is the main reason why FGAs are no longer popular. Psychiatrists have agonized about giving patients drugs that might cause it. Since the frequency of tardive dyskinesia is lower with second generation antipsychotics (Kane, 2004; Margolese *et al.*, 2005), most practitioners prefer them. Even so, since tardive dyskinesia is usually dose-dependent (Margolese *et al.*, 2005), many patients can be maintained on low-dose FGAs with minimal risk.

4.2   SECOND GENERATION ANTIPSYCHOTICS

Atypical antipsychotics, also called second generation antipsychotics (SGAs), have become the standard drugs for managing schizophrenia and the other psychoses. The first SGA to be introduced, in the 1960s, was clozapine (Wahlbeck, Cheine, and Essali, 2007). The drug had been withdrawn because of dangerous side effects (agranulocytosis), but eventually returned to the market as an agent designed for treatment-resistant schizophrenia. Clozapine even became something of a media celebrity. It was hailed as a miracle drug on the cover of *Time Magazine* (July 6, 1992). Experience since then shows that not every patient responds to clozapine, but it is still used for difficult cases with resistant schizophrenia, accompanied by careful blood monitoring (Wahlbeck, Cheine, and Essali 1997).

Some experts (Meltzer *et al.*, 2003) consider clozapine to be underutilized, given the evidence that it may reduce the high rate of suicide in schizophrenia, estimated to be about 5% (Inskip, Harris, and Barraclough, 1998). But as with all research on suicide prevention, it is difficult to determine whether clozapine actually prevents patients from killing themselves. The problem is that compliance with treatment, as well as close follow-up for hematological monitoring, could reduce that risk. The conclusion of one large-scale study (Alphs *et al.*, 2004) was that prospective data and randomization are needed to answer this question.

Another line of argument suggesting that clozapine may be underutilized comes from mortality data. In an 11-year follow-up of patients with schizophrenia, Tiihonen *et al.* (2009) found that the risk of early death was significantly lower in patients given this drug than it was for other atypicals. Thus the benefit to patients outweighed any risk of blood dyscrasia. This raises the question as to whether clozapine should become a first-line treatment (Kerwin, 2007). At this point, as suggested by the NICE guidelines (2009), it remains a back-up option for patients who do not respond to other atypicals.

In the last 15 years, two "blockbuster" SGAs have dominated the market: risperidone and olanzapine. Risperidone is rather more like a FGA, and its main side effect, particularly in higher doses, is EPS. It is also available in a long-term injectable form for non-compliant patients. Olanzapine is chemically related to clozapine but does not seem to share all its advantages, or its side effects. This drug is less likely to cause EPS, but has, as we will see, serious metabolic effects.

The booming success of risperidone and olanzapine opened up a market for competitors. Quetiapine, a molecule from a different chemical group, became another "blockbuster" drug. It is indeed an effective antipsychotic (Srisurapanont, Maneeton, and Maneeton, 2004), with metabolic effects similar to olanzapine. But its wide prescription for off-label indications is another story.

Quetiapine has made a lot of money for its manufacturer. But all things must come to an end, and the patent on the drug has recently expired. This has led to the company using an all too common ploy: the drug has been re-marketed in a "sustained release" form.

Aripiprazole, a more recent entrant to the market, may not have the same metabolic effects as other atypicals (El-Sayeh *et al.*, 2004). Ziprasidone is an antipsychotic that has been on the market for about ten years, and it also has fewer metabolic effects than olanzapine or quetiapine (Nemeroff *et al.*, 2005). But thus far, probably due to concern about cardiotoxicity, it has not been widely prescribed.

Let us consider more closely the metabolic syndrome caused by SGAs. Weight gain is common, and that can lead to diabetic complications (Newcomer and Haupt, 2006). Although this problem can develop with any atypical, it is particularly common with olanzapine (Jayaram, Hosalli, and Stroup, 2006). Even if the syndrome does not progress to diabetes, obesity is a serious problem that interferes with general health and social adjustment. It is more difficult to rehabilitate psychotic patients who have just gained 30 pounds. Weight gain is also a strong reason to be cautious about the off-label use of SGAs.

In addition to metabolic syndrome, research has established that atypical antipsychotics are associated with increased mortality when prescribed to elderly patients with dementia (Lee *et al.*, 2004; Schneider, Dagerman, and Insel, 2005). All SGAs now have a blackbox warning from the FDA warning against their use in the elderly. Psychiatrists and primary care physicians working with demented patients should look at other options for sedation. There is also an increased risk of sudden death associated with antipsychotics in middle-aged patients (Ray *et al.*, 2009). As has happened so many times in the history of medicine, some of the most serious side effects of drugs only become apparent after years of use.

4.3   ARE ATYPICALS BETTER THAN TYPICALS?

There are many reasons for the popularity of atypicals, but increased efficacy against psychosis is not one of them. These drugs are no more effective than typicals for patients with schizophrenia.

For many years, industry worked hard to convince psychiatrists that SGAs were superior. As older drugs went out of patent, the newer agents were marketed aggressively. One idea, presented at many CME conferences I have attended, was that SGAs had the capacity to reduce negative symptoms. That claim turned out not to be true (Murphy *et al.*, 2006). Confusion arose because controlling positive symptoms could look like an improvement in negative symptoms. Yet there was never any evidence than these drugs are effective for reversing the social withdrawal and apathy seen in chronic schizophrenia. These deficits seem to be an intrinsic characteristic of the disease process, associated with structural changes in the brain (Williamson, 2006).

The question as to whether atypicals are more efficacious than typicals in controlling the symptoms of schizophrenia has been addressed in detail in two large-scale multi-site studies (Foussias and Remington, 2010). The first, based at several US universities, was the Clinical Antipsychotic Trials of Antipsychotic Effectiveness (CATIE). The second, led by a group of British researchers, was the Cost Utility of the Latest Antipsychotic Drugs in Schizophrenia Study (CUtLASS-1). The results of both studies dispelled any notion of superiority for atypicals. (It is worth noting that both these trials were funded by government agencies – not by industry – and that most of the researchers involved were quite surprised by the findings.)

CATIE (Lieberman *et al.*.., 2005) randomized schizophrenic patients to treatment with olanzapine (7.5–30 mg qd), perphenazine (8–32 mg qd), quetiapine (200–800 mg qd), risperidone (1.5–6.0 mg qd), or ziprasidone (40–160 mg qd). This was an effectiveness trial not an RCT, and there was no blinding. In addition, treating physicians were allowed to add antiParkinsonian agents to combat EPS, and patients were allowed to make choices about alternatives if they did not remit with a given therapy. We already knew from previous RCTs that all these drugs are efficacious, but the CATIE study found no differences in effectiveness for any of the options it examined. Thus none of the SGAs was superior to the "golden oldie" FGA perphenazine.

CUtLASS (Jones *et al.*, 2006) used a different design, randomizing FGAs against SGAs, but allowing clinicians to choose the specific agent. Yet again, no difference was found between FGAs and SGAs, either for symptoms or for quality of life. Notably, clozapine outperformed the other SGAs. (Again, one has to ask whether this drug is under-prescribed.)

An editorial review co-authored by the leaders of both projects (Lewis and Lieberman, 2008) was entitled: "Can We Handle the Truth?" The authors described the implications as follows (p. 263):

> Our conclusion must be that first-generation drugs, if carefully pre-scribed, are as good as most second-generation drugs in many if not most patients with established schizophrenia. This is good news as it increases the range of choices of antipsychotic drugs. Care-ful prescribing of first-generation antipsychotics means using lower doses than was often done in the past and avoiding high-potency drugs. Clozapine clearly remains an important drug where others have failed.

The very same conclusion emerged in a recent large-scale meta-analysis (Leucht, Kissling, and Davis, 2009). In a comment on that paper, Tyrer and Kendall (2009, p. 1592) concluded:

> The only second-generation antipsychotic that is obviously better than other drugs in resistant schizophrenia is clozapine, and this is a very old drug indeed.

In summary, atypicals do not do anything for schizophrenia that typicals cannot. Side effect profiles are different but not better. Psy-chiatrists might consider returning to prescribing FGAs – particularly piperazine phenothiazines. They are cheaper and have favorable side effect profiles. The only substantive reason for prescribing the SGAs is the avoidance of tardive dyskinesia. Yet as Lewis and Lieberman (2008) note, the risk can be minimized by keeping doses low.

From the point of view of cost, even a partial return to FGAs would have a dramatic impact. Patients, as well as insurance companies, hospitals, and governments, would save large sums if physicians did not routinely prescribe expensive new drugs.

4.4 ANTIPSYCHOTICS IN MOOD DISORDERS

There are three strongly evidence-supported indications for antipsy-chotics. In addition to schizophrenia, there is good data to support their use in bipolar disorder and in unipolar psychotic depression.

In bipolar disorder, antipsychotics were for many years the mainstay of management for acute mania, and they retain a role in an emergency situation. Antipsychotics work fast, while lithium can take a week or so to take effect. Moreover, RCTs show that full control of manic episodes often requires a combination of mood stabilizers and antipsychotics (Scherk, Pajonk, and Leucht, 2007).

However, it does not follow that all bipolar patients need dual therapy for maintenance. Without a secure method of identifying those who require two drugs, it makes sense to begin with monotherapy (a mood stabilizer) and add antipsychotics only when patients are not well controlled (Alda, 2009).

It has also long been established that neuroleptics can be needed to manage psychotic symptoms associated with severe depression. This conclusion was confirmed by a meta-analysis of studies on FGAs (Parker, Hadzi-Pavlovic, and Pedic, 1992), and for SGAs in the large-scale Study of Pharmacotherapy of Psychotic Depression (STOP-PD; Andreescu *et al.*, 2007).

Thus in both mania and depression, we use antipsychotics to treat psychotic symptoms, independent of diagnosis. In addition to their antipsychotic effects, these drugs add a needed level of sedation to the treatment of agitated patients. But the fact that SGAs are useful *adjunctive* agents in some types of mood disorder does not mean that antipsychotics should be classified as mood stabilizers or antidepressants. Those who have drawn that conclusion (e.g., Ghaemi *et al.*, 2008) are confusing secondary with primary effects. These drugs should not be first-line choices in either bipolar or unipolar disorders. They are adjuncts that can be considered when symptoms are not controlled with other drugs.

Just how effective are antipsychotics as adjuncts in depression? A meta-analysis of 16 reports (Nelson and Papakostas, 2009), as well as a systematic review (Papakostas and Shelton, 2008), concluded that atypicals can be effective adjuncts to antidepressants in nonpsychotic treatment-resistant depression. However all these analyses were based on small samples with short durations of treatment, and all studies were industry-sponsored. We would need independently sponsored clinical trials in large and clinically representative samples with longer treatment to conclude that atypical antipsychotics are consistently effective.

We need more evidence before rushing ahead to offer atypical antipsychotics to patients who do not respond to antidepressants. Earlier reviewers of this literature (Nemeroff, 2005) had been skeptical about the state of the evidence, and one group (Shekelle *et al.*, 2007) concluded: "With few exceptions, there is insufficient high-grade evidence to reach conclusions about the efficacy of atypical antipsychotic medications for any of the off-label indications, either vs. placebo or vs. active therapy."

For better or for worse, the FDA has now approved two atypicals (aripiprazole and quetiapine) for the treatment of depression – to be used when antidepressants fail. The supporting evidence for aripiprazole was drawn from only two industry-funded studies (Berman, Marcus, and Swanink, 2007; Marcus, McQuade, and Carson, 2008), and Carroll (2009) has disputed the clinical significance of the data. In the case of quetiapine, only two studies (Cutler *et al.*, 2009; Weisler *et al.*, 2009) were used to support the indication, and both were funded by industry. Notably, since quetiapine has gone generic, these trials used the *sustained release* version, which remains on patent (Bauer *et al.*, 2009). Unfortunately, SGAs were not part of the STAR*D effectiveness study of treatment-resistant depression (see Chapter 6), nor have there been any meta-analyses taking unpublished RCT data into account.

The FDA has probably made a mistake in prematurely supporting an indication for SGAS in non-psychotic depression. We need more research, and since the side-effect burden of antipsychotics is considerable, we should be cautious about prescribing these drugs to depressed patients.

Meanwhile, there has been a large-scale advertising campaign for aripiprazole in the USA. One can hardly turn on the television without seeing these commercials, which feature an attractive woman (who has evidently recovered from her depression). Patients are told to ask their doctors "if this drug is right for you."

Advertisements for quetiapine have been more directed to physicians, and they promote the sustained release (i.e., still patented) version of the drug. If you read these advertisements, they acknowledge that quetiapine is not more effective than standard antidepressants, but suggest it be used in treatment-resistant cases. My concern is that given the large number of patients who do not respond well to standard antidepressants (see Chapter 6), this option could become routine.

Finally, we need to ask a separate question as to whether antipsychotics prevent the *recurrence* of mood disorders. There have been a few reports suggesting that they might have a preventive effect in mania, but these studies failed to follow patients long enough. For example, a report on olanzapine in bipolar disorder (Tohen *et al.*, 2006) only had a one-year follow-up. A study of quetiapine in bipolar disorder (Suppes *et al.*, 2009) looked at preventive effects over two years, but the sample was not representative. (Most potential subjects were either not entered into the study because they failed to respond to quetiapine in the acute phase, or dropped out in the course of follow-up.) As Chapter 5 will show, lithium remains the best option to prevent relapse of mania.

In summary, atypicals have a role to play in mania and depression, particularly when psychotic symptoms are prominent. We need to know more about when to prescribe them to non-psychotic patients. At this point the evidence is insufficient to support their use as primary agents for patients with mood disorders.

4.5 ATYPICAL USES FOR ATYPICAL NEUROLEPTICS

The title of this section comes from a review article (Brooke, Wiersgalla, and Salzman, 2005) which asked whether it makes sense to use drugs with such a serious side effect profile for "off-label" indications. Largely due to aggressive marketing, atypicals are being prescribed for a wide variety of symptoms that have little to do with psychosis.

The off-label use of drugs is rarely evidence-based. Yet there are no regulations preventing physicians from prescribing in any way they choose (Stafford, 2008).

Although no formal surveys have been published, my observation as a consultant has been that primary care physicians have been using SGAs widely for anxiety, mild depression, or insomnia. In particular, quetiapine is being prescribed as an anxiolytic, a hypnotic, and an antidepressant. The use of SGAs for these non-standard indications has to be questioned.

But why is quetiapine particularly popular? One reason may be that it has strong sedative properties. And it is perceived of as harmless. Evidently its metabolic side effects are not widely understood. (I see many patients who have significant weight gain after taking this drug). Moreover quetiapine is often given in high doses that would be suitable for psychotic patients, but not for garden-variety anxiety and depression.

In my own consultations on patients treated in primary care for depression and anxiety, many are already on antipsychotics. This practice may reflect marketing, over-enthusiasm, or both. If one is looking for sedation, benzodiazepines and SSRIs remain viable alternatives. For patients with mild to moderate depression, these drugs should not be a first choice. Even if they can be effective, I question their value for this purpose.

At this point, the off-label uses of antipsychotics are not based on solid evidence, but on open trials and clinical reports (Gao *et al.*, 2006; Brooke, Wiersgalla, and Salzman, 2005). And metabolic syndrome is in no way a minor problem. One should also keep tardive dyskinesia in mind. Since SGAs replaced haldoperidol, the problem is less talked about. But SGAs are also associated with *some* chance of causing tardive dyskinesia. That is an unnecessary risk to take in patients with mood disorders, unless there is a specific indication or necessity for the prescription (Keck *et al.*, 2000).

Even when one looks at the on-label use of antipsychotics, there are prescription practices I see that are less than rational. One is the use of multiple antipsychotics, a strategy that has never undergone clinical testing. Another is an over-use of injectable depot antipsychotics. Patients who will not take their medication, and who frequently relapse as a result, often need this regime. But I continue to see patients who are on a large number of oral meds *in addition* to injectables. If patients can be trusted to take other pills, why not prescribe oral antipsychotics?

In summary, when used for the purpose for which they were developed, antipsychotics are among the most consistently effective drugs in psychiatry. They are essential elements in the treatment of several major mental disorders. But their value in common mental disorders is doubtful.

CHAPTER 5

Mood Stabilizers and Mood Instability

Like antipsychotics, mood stabilizers are excellent drugs when used properly, but of doubtful value for off-label indications.

What is a mood stabilizer? Definitions of drug classes have real implications for practice. The idea that these agents have specific effects on mood instability has led them to be widely prescribed. Yet almost any sedating drug has the potential to damp down mood swings. Moreover, an agent that works that way in a specific category like bipolar disorder may not stabilize mood in other mental illnesses.

We also need to separate the short-term effects of mood stabilizers in manic or depressive episodes from their role in preventing recurrences. If *any* drug that can manage acute episodes of bipolar disorder were to be called a mood stabilizer, antipsychotics would fall in that class (a claim that has indeed been made). But if we were to restrict the definition to drugs proven to prevent recurrences of bipolar disorder, the only fully proven mood stabilizer is lithium. To avoid confusion, the NICE guidelines (National Institute for Clinical Excellence, 2006) refuse to use the term "mood stabilizer," favoring the more precise alternative "antimanic." Lithium, as well as the anti-epileptic drugs that are now used for the same indications, have well-established anti-manic effects, and can sometimes be useful for bipolar depression.

Whether these agents stabilize mood in patients with non-bipolar diagnoses is another question entirely. Mania is not the same as affective instability, in which mood changes rapidly in response to environmental stimuli. It remains to be proven whether mood stabilizers are useful for such symptoms (Paris, 2009).

5.1 CLASSIC INDICATIONS FOR MOOD STABILIZERS

Lithium was a miracle drug. Its introduction into practice was one of the greatest moments in the history of psychiatry. After being discovered in Australia (and then languishing in obscurity for almost two decades), lithium was eventually, and successfully, introduced into practice (Baastrup and Schou, 1967). I was in training at the time, and will never forget the results I witnessed in patients who previously had been unmanageable. Some who had been admitted ten or 20 times were stabilized and never hospitalized again.

Anticonvulsants form the bulk of the other mood stabilizers. These agents are also useful, but have less dramatic effects. And patients who cannot tolerate lithium may benefit from these agents.

There are several clinical scenarios in which mood stabilizers have been shown to be effective. As discussed in Chapter 4, acute manic episodes in bipolar disorder can be controlled with antipsychotics. But lithium has a more specific effect and has been shown to prevent recurrences. That is the main reason why it was a breakthrough.

Even today, nothing works quite as well as lithium. Unfortunately, this drug can have serious side effects. The most frequent are polydypsia and polyuria and hypothyroidism; one occasionally sees reduction of glomerular function (Goodwin and Jamieson, 2007). Fortunately not all patients suffer from these side effects. And in spite of its drawbacks, there are two reasons why lithium remains the first choice for most patients with bipolar-I disorder. First, it prevents recurrences of mania better than any existing alternatives (Ghaemi, Soldani, and Hsu, 2003). Second, lithium therapy seems to lower the rate of suicide in bipolar patients (Goodwin *et al.*, 2003). It is possible that this may not be a direct effect, if patients who *comply* with lithium therapy are less likely to complete suicide. This relationship has been confirmed in prospective trials (Cipriani, Barbul, and Geddes, 2005; Baldessarini *et al.*, 2006). It has even been reported that communities with more lithium in drinking water have a lower suicide rate (Ohgami *et al.*, 2009).

Why then have alternative mood stabilizers, developed as anticonvulsants, so often been preferred to lithium? One reason is that a natural salt like lithium has never been a money-maker for industry. Another is that the newer drugs have more favorable side effect profiles. They may be preferred when lithium's side effects are problematic, or when illness is less severe. Thus, although not as effective for maintenance, anticonvulsants tend to be preferred in bipolar-II disorder, in which the consequences of a recurrence are less catastrophic.

The first anticonvulsant mood stabilizer, carbamazepine, has not been popular, mainly because it tends to produce agranulocytosis – a danger that requires careful monitoring (Daughton, Padala, and Gabel, 2006). Valproate, a much less toxic drug, is more widely prescribed. While there are several other mood stabilizers (topiramate, gabapentin, and lamotrigine), valproate has the largest body of research behind it, and there is evidence that it can control acute mania (Bowden *et al.*, 1994; Bowden, 2007).

To determine whether anticonvulsants prevent recurrences of mania, one would need to follow patients over long periods. This kind of research is very rare. While older studies had suggested that lithium is a preventive against relapse, prospective research was needed. One large-scale report (Bowden *et al.*, 2000) failed to find *any* preventive effect for either valproate or lithium. But it only followed its cohort for 12 months, not long enough to assess relapse prevention. A study by Tondo, Baldessarini, and Floris (2001) confirmed the effectiveness of maintenance lithium therapy when bipolar-I and bipolar-II patients were followed for a mean of 8.3 years.

Meta-analyses have confirmed that lithium is the drug with the best evidence for maintenance (Geddes *et al.*, 2004). A Cochrane report (Macritchie *et al.*, 2001) concluded that valproate, in spite of its effectiveness for acute mania, has *not* been shown to be effective in preventing recurrence. A recent large-scale trial confirmed this verdict, although it also suggested that some patients do better with a combination of lithium and valproate (Geddes, 2010). Once again there is good reason to make lithium a first choice. Unfortunately, not all bipolar patients are given the benefit of this option.

Lamotrigine has been approved by the FDA as a maintenance drug, on the basis of an 18-month follow-up in which it produced results comparable to lithium (Bowden *et al.*, 2003). However, this conclusion was rather premature, since it lacked longer follow-up and/or replication. Moreover, the study on which the recommendation was made was industry-funded.

Another common maintenance strategy is to add an atypical neuroleptic to the mood stabilizer. We have seen that this combination is often required for acute management (Chapter 4). However, as emphasized by Alda (2009), and supported by a recent Cochrane report (Cipriani *et al.*, 2009), the evidence for lithium monotherapy as a preventive is stronger than for any combination with antipsychotics.

In summary, if a patient has bipolar-I disorder, there are a number of options for acute treatment, but lithium should usually be the first choice. If a patient has bipolar-II disorder, lithium is also the best documented option (Hadjipavlou and Yatham, 2008), although one can choose to prescribe a less toxic mood stabilizer.

To optimize the treatment of bipolar disorders, the National Institute of Mental Health (NIMH) initiated the Systematic Treatment Enhancement Program for Bipolar Disorder (STEP-BD). Its goals were to follow a large group of patients so as to determine optimal treatment. One of its main findings was that patients are likely to relapse unless they become *fully* asymptomatic (Judd *et al.*, 2008), a goal that is difficult to achieve. But the STEP-BD program only followed patients for two years, limiting the generalizability of these results.

Both bipolar-I and bipolar-II patients may spend more time feeling low than high. A large literature on *bipolar depression* has emerged, a term referring to patients who have had manic or hypomanic episodes, and then become depressed (Parker, 2000, 2008). STEP-BD found that adding paroxetine or bupropion to mood stabilizers in bipolar depression is not effective, and recovery difficult to achieve, with subsyndromal symptoms or full relapse being very common (Parikh, LeBlanc, and Ovanessian, in press). A recent meta-analysis confirmed that antidepressants are not consistently effective for bipolar depression, and that atypical neuroleptics are also not very effective (Ghaemi *et al.*, 2008). While some authorities (Young, 2008) conclude that mood stabilizers remain the main treatment for bipolar depression, STEP-BD (Nierenberg *et al.*, 2006) reported only equivocal effects. Clearly this clinical picture is unusually difficult to treat.

There has long been concern about the possibility that antidepressants can "flick the switch" from depression into mania. Patients who switch from depression to mania when treated with antidepressants have sometimes been described as having a "bipolar-III" disorder (Ghaemi, Ko, and Goodwin, 2002).

Actually that scenario turns out to be rare, and our level of worry about it has probably been excessive (Parker and Parker, 2003). It is possible that switching was something of a clinical myth, originally derived from case reports, and passed on from generation to generation, but never confirmed by systematic research. Part of the confusion arises from the fact that many bipolar patients initially present with depressive symptoms. When mania develops, clinicians may attribute the change to the antidepressant that they have just prescribed. But the switch may have happened with or without treatment – bipolar disorder may simply be running its course.

In summary, psychiatry can be proud of having effective drugs to stabilize mood in patients with classical bipolar disorders. Lithium remains the gold standard for prevention of recurrence. The popularity of anticonvulsant mood stabilizers is only partially justified.

5.2 WHAT IS BIPOLARITY?

The concept of bipolar disorders has broadened, and the idea of a broad spectrum of conditions, all of which might require similar treatment, has created a major controversy (Paris, 2009). Under the influence of prominent specialists in the field (Akiskal, 2002; Angst and Gamma, 2002), physicians have been encouraged to make this diagnosis much more readily. But before deciding what to treat, and how to treat, we need to know what bipolarity is and what it is not.

Kraepelin (1921) famously divided the psychoses into two groups: dementia praecox (later renamed schizophrenia), and manic-depression (later renamed bipolar disorder). The basic concept of bipolar mood disorder, retained in DSM-IV-TR and ICD-10, is of a disabling illness with clearcut manic episodes. Today we call that clinical picture *bipolar-I*. Since full mania is likely to require admission to a ward, I hesitate to make this diagnosis in patients who have never been hospitalized.

The diagnostic problem is more complex in patients who meet criteria for *bipolar-II*. This category differs from bipolar-I in presenting with hypomanic rather than full manic episodes. Many of these patients have never required hospital admission.

The problem in bipolar-II concerns the definition of hypomania. The DSM-IV-TR definition is not equivalent to the presence of "mood swings." A hypomanic episode is a period in which mood is either "high" (elevated) or irritable. During this period, if mood is "high," a diagnosis of hypomania requires the presence of at least three out of seven symptoms persistently: grandiosity, decreased need for sleep, pressure of speech, flight of ideas or racing thoughts, distractibility, overactivity, and impulsive behaviors. But if mood is only irritable rather than elevated, then at least four of these same seven criteria are required. Crucially, these features must be present *continuously for at least four days*. In contrast, people who have mood swings will not be high or irritable for four days, but will shift around, often slipping back into depression (Koenigsberg, in press; Zimmerman *et al.*, 2008).

The criteria for hypomania, like most of those in DSM-IV-TR, are fairly arbitrary. But it seems better to be restrictive and con-servative than to expand a diagnosis without good reason. It has been suggested that DSM-V should drop the four-day rule, but that would be a mistake. Unfortunately, psychiatry has a long history of extending diagnostic constructs, such as schizophrenia or de-pression (Paris, 2008a). Bipolar illness is a meaningful diagnosis that has been studied for many decades – extending it can only dilute it.

Moreover, patients with clear-cut hypomania fall into a recogniz-able clinical entity that requires different treatment from bipolar-I (Hadjipavalou, Mok, and Latham, 2008). Unfortunately not all clini-cians apply (or remember) the standard criteria for hypomania when diagnosing bipolar-II. Mood swings of any kind tend to lead to a knee-jerk response. In my consultation practice, I often see patients referred for a putative diagnosis of bipolarity who have shown nothing more than moodiness.

The shift in diagnostic practice for bipolar disorder has also had a profound impact on the general public. The idea that one is bipolar (or more likely, that someone else in the family is) has become common. Since so many people have unstable mood, the idea that it is a disorder that can be treated with drugs is appealing. I often consult on patients who have made a self-diagnosis and who are specifically looking for treatment with a mood stabilizer.

There is no doubt that bipolar disorder was under-diagnosed in the past, especially in North America. Four decades ago, researchers observed that US psychiatrists were diagnosing schizophrenia in patients whom British psychiatrists considered to be manic-depressive (Cooper, Kendell, and Gurland, 1972). It later became apparent that features considered "typical" of schizophrenia were actually frequent in bipolar patients (Abrams and Taylor, 1981). With time, US psychiatrists fell into line with their British colleagues, and actively embraced the concept of bipolarity – even more closely than their counterparts in the UK. (Is this another example of Americans "rushing off madly in all directions?")

The preference for seeing psychotic patients as bipolar was greatly influenced by the success of lithium therapy. Psychiatrists wanted to make a diagnosis that could lead to effective treatment and that seemed to be associated with a better prognosis. Within a few years, a wide range of patients had their diagnosis changed from schizophrenia, and were prescribed lithium. It was correctly pointed out that some of these patients had bipolar relatives, and that lithium responders could be found among patients with "first-order Schneiderian symptoms," then thought to be typical of schizophrenia (Abrams and Taylor, 1981). I saw several patients rediagnosed with bipolar-I disorder in that era who, after being put on lithium, had no further relapses. For almost the first time in the history of psychiatry, diagnosis really made a difference.

However, I also observed a tendency for my colleagues to interpret *any* degree of mood disturbance as a sign of bipolarity, and an indication for a change of drugs to provide patients with "the benefit of lithium." Patients with schizophrenia can have periods of depression, and when agitated, have symptoms that are difficult to differentiate from manic excitement. And since psychosis is a fluctuating illness, making it difficult to define what is and what is not a drug effect, many patients who were given lithium (to see if they could benefit from it) stayed on the drug long-term.

This was the beginning of a love affair between American psychiatry and bipolar illness. With time, the love of mania became a mania in its own right (Healy, 2009).

The next step in the expansion of the bipolar concept was also stimulated by drug development. As long as lithium was the main treatment option, its toxicity did not greatly encourage practitioners to make a bipolar diagnosis. But newer mood stabilizers (as well as atypical neuroleptics), even if less effective than lithium for mania and hypomania, were better tolerated by patients.

Dissenters continue to think that bipolarity should retain its classic definition, in order to better define a treatment response. Alda (1999) has argued that lithium-responsive patients should be put into a different diagnostic category from those who do not respond to lithium. In support of this view, Alda reported genetic variations related to lithium-responsiveness that are not shared with lithium-unresponsive populations.

In contrast, other researchers on bipolar disorders have advocated a shift from the classical concept of illness to a very broad spectrum. This process seems to be a universal tendency in psychiatry. Every research group seems to want to expand its definition and increase the frequency of diagnosis. (I bend over backwards to avoid doing that for my own area of research, personality disorders).

The bipolar spectrum was a powerful idea that seemed to explain much that had long remained obscure. But in the long run, the story may reflect the aphorism of the nineteenth century British biologist Thomas Huxley, who described the tragedy of "*a beautiful theory slain* by an ugly fact." Let us examine some of these facts.

5.3   THE BIPOLAR SPECTRUM

Ghaemi, Ko, and Goodwin (2002) published a review article summarizing the views of those who favor a broader spectrum. The authors suggested that bipolarity can take four basic forms: *bipolar I*, the classical manic-depressive diagnosis described by Kraepelin; *bipolar II*, depression with spontaneous hypomanic episodes; *bipolar III*, in which hypomanic episodes occur only as a result of taking antidepressants; and *bipolar IV*, an "ultra-rapid-cycling" disorder in which mood swings occur on a daily or even hourly basis.

Kraepelin (1921) had allowed for a spectrum of milder conditions that did not meet the full (and usually psychotic) picture that brought patients into hospital. However, he never claimed that mood swings of any kind are a sub-clinical form of hypomania. Nor did he envisage a bipolar spectrum affecting a large spectrum of the general population.

Ghaemi *et al.* (2002) would diagnose rapid mood instability as "bipolar-IV disorder." But we do not know whether such mood swings are in the same class as hypomanic episodes. One way out, as we have seen, would be to change the definition of hypomania. One of the more radical suggestions came from Benazzi (2004), who, based on a factor analysis of symptoms in bipolar-II, recommended a definition that would not even require a change in mood, but depend only on periods of overactivity.

Another way to extend the spectrum would be to remove any distinction between mood shifts that last an hour and those that last four days or more. Perugi and Akiskal (2002) have suggested that the four-day rule for diagnosing hypomania is mistaken, and should be redefined to include mood swings, whatever their duration.

In medicine, time scale has always been an important element in differential diagnosis. For example, patients are not considered to have essential hypertension if they reacted to an environmental stressor with a *temporary* rise in blood pressure. (That is why physicians routinely measure blood pressure several times in a row.) Diagnosis of a disease usually requires persistent change.

Instead of jumping to conclusions, one needs to establish the presence of hypomania by taking a careful history, as well as collecting observations from key informants. Only in this way can the clinician determine if there has been a *continuous* abnormality of mood over several days, not moodiness over a few hours.

Not following these rules can lead to clinical errors. For example, adolescents are famously moody (Susman and Rogol, 2004), but that does not mean they are often bipolar. Yet a recent survey in the US found that the diagnosis of bipolar disorder in adolescents and young adults has increased *fourfold* (Moreno *et al.*, 2007). Enthusiasts for the bipolar spectrum might argue that we are finally recognizing a serious problem. It seems more likely that we are looking at a diagnostic fad, as well as a treatment fad.

Akiskal (2002) has proposed a concept of "soft bipolarity," which he defines as a wide range of disturbances in mood, anxiety, or impulse control that fall within a spectrum. In a classical and more conservative framework, bipolarity had to be diagnosed by "hard" signs and symptoms. The "soft" concept reflects a search for patients for whom mood stabilizers would be prescribed.

But what if such symptoms are no more of a marker for any specific disease than inflammation or jaundice? The patients for whom mood stabilizers are being prescribed could well suffer from a heterogeneous group of conditions that do not respond to these drugs, and will not show the same response as in classical bipolar disorder.

Another point of confusion about the boundaries of bipolarity is *irritability* (excessive feelings of annoyance or frustration with a person or situation). It is well known that irritable mood sometimes dominates the clinical picture in full mania (Goodwin and Jamieson, 2007). But it has been proposed that irritability is a "soft" feature that can replace elevated mood as a criterion for hypomania (Akiskal, 2002). Needless to say, many people are irritable, for many reasons. It is hard to see how this trait is in any way specific to bipolar disorder.

Impulsivity (the tendency to act on the spur of the moment) is another feature that has been considered as a marker for bipolarity (Akiskal, 2002). Again, the presence of such a pattern does not point specifically to any diagnosis, since it is found in substance abuse, personality disorders, eating disorders, and many other diagnostic categories (Moeller et al., 2001).

A final point of confusion about the boundaries of bipolarity derives from the concept of "mixed states" of mania and depression (Akiskal and Benazzi, 2003). Unfortunately this is a slippery and inadequately researched concept. Mixed states have been used to describe all kinds of abnormal emotional reactions in patients who do not have consistently elevated mood.

Moreover, most of the features attributed to soft bipolarity are extremely common in the community. Once one interprets high prevalence behaviors of all kinds in this way, it is difficult to see how *anyone* can escape being called bipolar.

5.4 AFFECTIVE INSTABILITY

Mood instability, usually called affective instability (AI), is a different construct from bipolarity. It describes several inter-related phenomena: high intensity of emotional response, a slow rate of return to baseline, an excessive reactivity to psychosocial cues, and a tendency to switch rapidly from one mood to another (Koenigsberg *et al.*, 2002).

Mood swings usually last a few hours, or at most a day. While it has been suggested that "ultra-short" mood instability could be categorized as "bipolar-IV" disorder (Ghaemi *et al.*, 2002), this kind of affective instability is well known to be characteristic of personality disorders, especially the borderline category (Paris, 2008b).

The general definition of a personality disorder depends on a long-term dysfunction in work, relationships, and emotional regulation (American Psychiatric Association, 2000). That pattern stands in contrast to the episodic nature of mood disorders. While it has been claimed that personality disorders themselves are nothing but bipolar variants (Akiskal, 2004; Perugi and Akiskal, 2002), these conditions rarely evolve over time into bipolar illness (Paris, Gunderson, and Weinberg, 2007).

The bipolar spectrum concept assumes that all mood dysregulation lies on a continuum. But is also possible that the tendency to become irritable, sad, or too readily overexcited is a personality trait. Moreover, based on treatment response, affective instability and bipolarity are separate phenomena (Paris, Gunderson, and Weinberg, 2007). Clinical trials of mood stabilizers in patients with borderline personality disorder have been unimpressive (Paris, 2008c). Mood stabilizers do not produce a remission of personality disorders, as they so often do in classical bipolar illness (Paris, 2008c).

In the personality disorder literature, AI has also been described using the term *emotional dysregulation*, a pattern of strong and prolonged response to stressors (Linehan, 1993; Henry *et al.*, 2001; Koenigsberg *et al.*, 2002; Russell *et al.*, 2007; Koenigsberg, in press). Research shows that patients with personality disorders have a different pattern of mood instability than in those diagnosed with bipolar-II (Koenigsberg *et al.*, 2002). Instead of moving from depression to elation, patients go from depression to anger (and stay angry for a long time).

Affective instability reflects environmental sensitivity rather than the spontaneous variability that characterizes bipolar disorder. It is an abnormal response to life events. That is why mood can change by the hour. Patients with this picture can be happy in morning, sad in the afternoon, and angry in the evening. In contrast, when patients are manic, it is impossible to "bring them down." And when patients are severely depressed, nothing can cheer them up.

Affective instability does not, by itself, point to a diagnosis of bipolar disorder. I would be willing to change my mind about this issue if it could be shown that lithium, valproate, or other mood stabilizers are highly effective for these patients, and produce true remission. Thus far there is no evidence to support such a view (Patten and Paris, 2008).

We have no truly effective pharmacological treatments for patients with substance abuse, personality disorders, or eating disorders. Most of the evidence suggests that these disorders benefit most from specialized psychotherapy (see Chapter 9). Yet many psychiatrists prefer drug treatment to entering that foreign territory. One also wonders if they simply want to believe that patients can be treated with the same pharmacological armamentarium that proved so successful in classical bipolar disorders.

5.5   ESTABLISHING DIAGNOSTIC BOUNDARIES

Medicine as a whole has moved from syndromal classification to disease definitions based on an understanding of etiology and pathogenesis. Unfortunately, psychiatry lacks the data to take this step. But we need to be patient, and avoid rushing in with facile solutions that could prove wrong in practice.

In theory, psychiatry could use several methods to establish valid boundaries between mental disorders (Robins and Guze, 1970). The ideal would be to identify biological markers for specific diseases. However no one has ever found markers for major mental illnesses – not for mania, not for hypomania, and certainly not for the bipolar spectrum. Without that kind of data, we cannot assume that common symptoms are associated with common endophenotypes.

Even though biological markers remain obscure, clues can be drawn from other sources. One is family history. It is true that bipolar disorder in a first-degree relative should increase suspicion for the disease. But while it has been claimed that a positive history of bipolarity can be documented in patients with bipolar spectrum disorders (Akiskal and Benazzi, 2003), the supporting data were not based on the presence of diagnosable bipolar disorders. Instead, using "softer" criteria, relatives with irritability and moodiness are scored as having symptoms of "bipolar spectrum disorder" (Merikangas et al., 2007). One cannot make valid diagnoses of family members with this kind of retrospective, vague, and second-hand data. We need to directly interview first-degree relatives using systematic methods that assess bipolar disorders.

Another clue to diagnostic boundaries is a course of illness – the criterion that Kraepelin originally used to define manic-depression. Yet there are no data showing that patients with "soft" bipolarity eventually develop "hard" symptoms.

Still another clue is treatment response. If it could be shown that patients with soft symptoms respond to mood stabilizers, that kind of data would support the bipolar spectrum concept. But as we have seen, there is no such evidence.

As long as psychiatrists do not understand the etiology and pathogenesis of bipolar disorder, they are working in the dark. One can treat patients effectively without full understanding of disease. But the fact that psychotic patients were sedated in the past with barbiturates provided no insight whatsoever into the nature of their illness. Similarly, the widespread prescription of mood stabilizers has provided no useful information about the nature of bipolarity.

5.6 IMPLICATIONS FOR TREATMENT

The concept of a bipolar spectrum has the potential to radically transform psychiatry. If, as has been claimed by proponents of the spectrum, bipolar disorders are extremely common in the general population, and in clinical populations, then mood stabilizers might become the most important group of drugs in psychiatry. Using DSM-IV definitions, the American National Comorbidity Study Replication (Kessler et al., 2005a) found that bipolar-I and bipolar-II together have a community prevalence of about 2%. Together, these numbers make bipolarity much more common than schizophrenia. But figures go much higher when sub-clinical variants are included. Advocates of the spectrum concept have estimated the prevalence of bipolarity to be 6% (Judd and Akiskal, 2003), or even 8% (Pini *et al.*, 2005). Merikangas *et al.* (2007), using an instrument designed to determine the frequency of bipolar spectrum disorders, found that while bipolar-I had a prevalence of 1%, and bipolar II was 1.1%, when they added sub-threshold cases (assessed with a new instrument specifically designed for the purpose) an additional 2.4% met criteria. The problem, as already discussed, is that moodiness and irritability are common in non-clinical populations. Thus the method of this study begged the question of what kind of phenomena truly lie within a bipolar spectrum. If what they were actually measuring was personality traits, characteristics that have long been known to run in families (Plomin *et al.*, 2001).

If one applies the spectrum concept to clinical populations, one sees even more elevated rates. In a large clinical sample in France, 39% of *all* patients were found to meet criteria (Akiskal *et al.*, 2006). One must wonder who the other 61% were – or did the researchers miss something?

If over a third of all psychiatric patients are bipolar, who are they? Most have traditionally received other diagnoses – including personality disorders, substance abuse, adult ADHD, and eating disorders (Akiskal, 2002; Angst and Gamma, 2002). Considering them as bipolar would lead us to treat most of these patients with mood stabilizers. This is already happening – in my experience as a consultant, I see many patients with such problems who have been prescribed an anticonvulsant or lithium.

In spite of these reservations, there is one group in which a substantive argument can be made for extending the range of bipolarity. Some unipolar depressions will evolve with time into bipolarity (Akiskal *et al.*, 2002). A family history of bipolar disorder, as well as the presence of psychosis, can help predict this outcome (Goodwin and Jamison, 2007). Even so, these are statistical relationships, and there is no basis in clinical practice for making accurate predictions of course in unipolar patients – or for prematurely offering mood stabilizers.

It is more of a stretch to claim that addictions, even if they are associated with prominent mood instability and loss of impulse control, fall within a bipolar spectrum (Maremanni *et al.*, 2004). While many bipolar patients suffer from substance abuse, it does not follow that substance abuse proves the presence of bipolarity, or that the "real" reason for using drugs lies in mood instability.

Similarly, the idea that substance abuse, eating disorders, and personality disorders (all characterized by impulsivity) reflect the bipolarity is based on reverse logic. It does not follow that since bipolar patients can be impulsive, patients with impulsive symptoms must be bipolar. Once again, signs and symptoms cannot be assumed to reflect valid diagnostic boundaries. Phenomenological resemblances do not prove common pathological mechanisms, or justify common methods of treatment.

I have called the idea that so many different forms of pathology are due to unstable mood *bipolar imperialism* (Paris, 2009). Accepting this principle would mean that nearly half of psychiatry is really about bipolarity, and it would lead to the prescription of mood stabilizers (as well as atypical neuroleptics) to half of our patients. Yet RCTs have not determined whether such practices are justified (Patten and Paris, 2008). Even so, as Chapter 7 will show, many patients today are receiving a cocktail of mood stabilizers, neuroleptics, antidepressants, and benzodiazepines. (This practice is sometimes described as "expert psychopharmacology.")

None of this should be interpreted as denying that mood stabilizers (and atypical neuroleptics) can be helpful for some non-bipolar patients. But these are sedative drugs – barbiturates did much the same thing in the past. The question is whether effects are in any way specific, and whether, in view of the toxicity of the drugs under question, they constitute the best choices.

5.7 CONCLUSIONS

Mood stabilizers are effective drugs that are being used in conditions for which they were not designed. At the same time, conditions that have never been considered to be forms of bipolarity are being redefined as such, and treated with drugs designed for classical bipolar illness.

As is the case for so many mental disorders, we do not know whether bipolar disorder is one disease or many. One cannot answer such a question by examining symptoms alone. Yet deciding where to draw the boundary has profound implications for practice. The concept of a broad bipolar spectrum is a radical idea that should not be put into clinical practice without very strong evidence.

The history of psychiatry has been marked by effective treatments that became ineffective when they were too widely applied. We need not repeat this story for mood stabilizers.

CHAPTER 6

Antidepressants

Antidepressants, like so many other drugs in psychiatry, are valuable agents that are frequently overprescribed. We now know that their effects on depression are not as consistent as previously believed. The problem seems to lie with an overly broad definition of what depression is. Sometimes antidepressants yield miraculous results. But they may do little but "take the edge off." And they sometimes do not work at all.

Antidepressants are also misnamed. In some ways, these drugs resemble Aspirin – they lower psychic pain but do not reverse underlying disease processes. Thus, while they have effects on mood, antidepressants are also useful for a wide range of other conditions. The list includes most anxiety disorders: panic, generalized anxiety, obsessive-compulsive disorder, and post-traumatic stress disorder (Scott, Davidson, and Palmer, 2001). Above and beyond mood and anxiety, antidepressants have also been useful for reducing impulsivity, as shown by RCTs in bulimia nervosa (Morgan, 2002; Bond, 2005) and in borderline personality disorder (Paris, 2008c).

Antidepressants have such a wide spectrum of action that they might be better called "antineurotics." They can reduce many symptoms, but effects are not disease-specific. This was nicely shown by a study in which an antidepressant (paroxetine) had distinct effects in depressed patients in reducing self-reported traits of *neuroticism* (Tang *et al.*, 2009). That dimension of personality measures reactivity to environmental events, and high levels are a diathesis for a very wide range of psychological symptoms.

The Use and Misuse of Psychiatric Drugs: An Evidence-Based Critique   by Joel Paris
© 2010 John Wiley & Sons, Ltd

6.1   DEFINING THE BOUNDARIES OF DEPRESSION

Depression is a heterogenous concept. Lowered mood can be a symptom, a syndrome, or a disorder.

Depression is so prevalent that it has sometimes been called "the common cold of psychiatry." But a cold should not be confused with pneumonia, even if both share some of the same pathological mechanisms. And treating colds as if they were pneumonia (i.e., with antibiotics) is just as mistaken as giving antidepressants to everyone whose mood is low. Calling different things by the same name lies at the root of many clinical problems.

Most people experience depressed feelings at some time during their lives. That need not mean they are suffering from a mental disorder. The broad concept of depression used in contemporary psychiatry fails to make these distinctions. It conflates normal unhappiness with the mental paralysis of melancholia (Parker, 2009; Horwitz and Wakefield; 2007).

DSM-IV-TR (American Psychiatric Association, 2000) and ICD-10 definition (World Health Organization, 1992) use similar criteria to define clinical depression. In DSM, a "major depressive episode" requires that patients meet five of nine listed criteria for a minimum of two weeks. That rather short time scale is a source of over-diagnosis in non-clinical populations. In patient samples, most people we see will have been ill for longer. A more serious problem is the soft nature of the other criteria. It is not clear where the number "five" came from, or whether it constitutes a valid cutoff point for pathology (Kendler and Gardner, 1998).

Moreover, it is fairly easy to meet five criteria for depression. One need only have a low mood, loss of interest or pleasure, and loss of energy, as well as reduced concentration – and four criteria are already met. Add to that either feelings of worthlessness, insomnia, weight loss, or suicidal thoughts, and the diagnosis is made. Transitory mood states related to environmental stressors, if they last for a couple of weeks, can easily produce such a picture.

This definition of major depression does not specifically exclude symptoms that occur primarily in response to obvious environmental stressors. DSM-IV-TR allows for the exclusion of extended periods of symptomatic distress following bereavement, but does not apply that rule to other losses. Yet a community study showed that depressive symptoms do not differ, whether caused by bereavement or by other life stressors (Wakefield *et al.*, 2007).

Surprisingly little research exists to validate the nine DSM criteria. In a twin study, Kendler and Gardner (1998) examined whether future depressive episodes (in either twin) could be predicted from an initial one. Their conclusions (p. 172) are worth quoting:

> The authors found little empirical support for the DSM-IV requirements for 2 weeks' duration, five symptoms, or clinically significant impairment. Most functions appeared continuous. These results suggest that major depression – as articulated by DSM-IV – may be a diagnostic convention imposed on a continuum of depressive symptoms of varying severity and duration.

In this light, epidemiological research based on the current DSM definition of major depression is suspect. These criteria inflate prevalence by including mild cases that do not necessarily require medical treatment (Patten, 2008). The lifetime prevalence of major depression in the National Comorbidity Survey, a large-scale US epidemiological study that used DSM-IV criteria, was 16.6% (Kessler *et al.*, 2005a). This high rate would have been reduced if a narrower definition had been used, and if symptoms arising from stressors that occur normally had been excluded (Wakefield *et al.*, 2007).

Diagnostic problems have clinical implications. If depression is too readily diagnosed, then the value of screening programs in the community is questionable, since this procedure is likely to identify cases that do not require treatment (Thombs *et al.*, 2008). There seems little justification to place research assistants in shopping malls to offer screening questionnaires for depression to passing visitors. Few of these potential patients will need antidepressants (even if that kind of therapy is most likely to be prescribed).

The difficulty in separating clinical states of depression from unhappiness should not be surprising. After all, life need not necessarily be happy. Even Sigmund Freud (1896/1957) once remarked that all that psychoanalysis aimed to do was "to turn neurotic misery into normal human unhappiness."

Diagnostic categories should be based on unique pathological processes. But there are no biological markers to validate the boundaries of depression. This diagnosis need not lead to any specific treatment.

Younger psychiatrists may not realize that until a few decades ago, there was no such diagnosis as "major depression." Depression has been defined rather differently from one era to the next. The present coinage arises from a *specific theory* about mood disorders – that all depressions lie on a continuum.

In the era when most psychiatrists worked in mental hospitals, the favored term for severe depression was *melancholia*. We can still recognize that clinical picture – and it is one of the few psychiatric conditions that resembles a medical disease (Parker and Manicavasagar, 2005).

The diagnosis of melancholia dates back to Hippocrates. It describes a condition lasting weeks to months in which patients suffer from despondency, irritability, and restlessness, with a slowing down of mental processes and movement, diminished appetite, sleeplessness, and powerful suicidal urges.

It is important to recognize melancholia because it requires different treatment. As we will see later in the chapter, antidepressants are more effective in these cases than in milder depressions. Melancholia often requires neuroleptic treatment, and it has a specific (and often gratifying) response to electroconvulsive therapy (Parker, 2005).

In contrast, "major depressive disorder" in DSM-IV-TR is very heterogeneous. It might best be considered a syndrome, not a medical diagnosis (Parker and Manicavasagar, 2005). It mixes the apples of melancholia with the oranges of mild, normative episodes of lower mood – and everything between. Healy (2009) has spoken of the *creation* of major depression, noting that this condition is not necessarily "major."

The authors of DSM-III had at one point considered introducing a category of "minor depression" that would be less severe and require different treatment (Shorter, 2009). But in the end, both DSM and ICD only allowed additional codes for severity within a broader diagnosis of major depression. Patients with transient depressive symptoms can also be diagnosed with "adjustment disorder with depressed mood" if they do not reach the bar of five out of nine criteria over two weeks. Patients with chronic but sub-clinical symptoms can be diagnosed with "dysthymia" if they have only two depressive criteria (with symptoms present most of the time over a two-year period). Dysthymia is not well researched, and it seems to be a combination of milder mood disorders and depressed symptoms that are frequently associated with other diagnoses (Klein and Santiago, 2003).

The conceptual basis for a major depressive episode is a broad and unitary model of depression. Some years before DSM-III was published, Akiskal and McKinney (1973) wrote an influential article arguing that older distinctions between depressive neurosis and psychotic depression were not valid, and that all types lie on a continuum. They noted that previous editions of DSM had attempted to make distinctions on the basis of unproven etiological theories (i.e., that neurotic depression was environmental while "endogenous," that is, melancholic depression was biological). DSM-III took up this point of view, and the unitary theory became a conventional wisdom.

Given the absence of clear cut-off points, there is some justification to viewing depression in a dimensional framework. However the unitary theory fails to deal with the two ends of the continuum. It does not acknowledge the uniqueness of melancholia, and it does not separate unhappiness from mental disorder.

The practical effect of the unitary theory was that it primed physicians to treat almost all depressed patients with drugs. As pharmacological treatment came to dominate the management of mood disorders, patients with milder symptoms were given antidepressants. Only recently has it become clear that this practice is not firmly evidence-based.

The DSM manual was not intended to be a guide to treatment. In fact, it has explicitly denied that implication, emphasizing that diagnoses are intended only as a common language for practice. It is not logical to assume that drug treatment follows from diagnosis.

The idea of specific diseases leading to specific therapies is deeply rooted in medicine. We see this in the way that drugs are approved for specific "indications," that is, DSM diagnoses (valid or not). Over time, these categories became reified, and psychiatrists have forgotten how they were "created."

Many physicians today think they would be remiss *not* to offer pharmacotherapy for depression. This attitude persists, even though psychotherapy has known for decades to be equally effective, at least in mild to moderate cases (Klerman *et al.*, 1974; Elkin *et al.*, 1989; Smith, Glass, and Miller, 1980).

We now know that when antidepressants are prescribed, less than half of depressions fully remit (Kirsch *et al.*, 2008). But a large body of research shows that severe depressions respond better to drugs than mild depressions (Parker, 2009). The severity issue is crucial. Over 20 years ago, a large-scale multi-site study in the US (Elkin *et al.*, 1989) found imipramine to be only marginally superior to a placebo (checkup) condition for mild depression. Yet the drug was definitely superior to both placebo and to psychotherapy in more severe depressions. Somehow this important lesson was lost over time with our tendency to treat every case in the same way.

Meta-analyses of research on modern antidepressants also show that drugs are superior in severe depression because placebo effects are weak, but are less efficacious when placebo effects are strong, as they are in "garden-variety" depressions (Kirsch *et al.*, 2008). Very similar findings emerged from a meta-analysis by Fournier *et al.* (2010) examining studies of imipramine and paroextine, in which drugs were found to be most effective in severe depression.

Parker (2009) emphasizes that the main reason why drugs are not always better than placebo derives from a failure to make diagnostic distinctions. These observations present a strong challenge to the unitary theory of depression. We need a classification that can predict, at least to some extent, which patients are most likely to respond to drug therapy. At this point, we do not have the data to do so.

6.2   OLDER ANTIDEPRESSANTS

Tricyclics were the first group of antidepressants to be widely prescribed (Monoamine oxidase inhibitors had been discovered first, but were never popular). Tricyclics are highly effective, but are not often used today.

As we have seen, physicians tend to prefer newer to older drugs. There is no doubt that newer agents have been heavily marketed. Moreover, tricyclics had real problems that made them unpopular. As compared to SSRIs, they are unpleasant to take. Anticholinergic side effects (dry mouth, blurred vision, and trouble urinating) are troublesome, and neither patients nor physicians ever felt fully comfortable with them. Moreover, overdose with a tricylic is dangerous.

Suicide attempts can be fatal with as little as one gram of imipramine, that is, a week's supply (Hirschfeld, 1999).

These are the main reasons why a newer generation of drugs almost entirely replaced tricylics. Many younger psychiatrists have no experience at all with the older agents. Selective serotonin reuptake inhibtors (SSRIs) have the advantage of greater tolerability and safety. If you want to be sure that your patient will actually take what you prescribe, you are generally better off prescribing an SSRI. The only problem is that these drugs do not always work.

Are tricylics better than SSRIs? Some say so, but the evidence is unclear. What we can conclude is that newer antidepressants are no more effective than older ones. In a meta-analysis of 11 comparative studies between tricylics and SSRIs carried out in primary care settings, MacGillivray *et al.* (2003) found no difference between these alternatives. It therefore makes sense to prefer drugs with a more favorable side effect profile.

Even so, it remains possible that tricyclics are better for *severe* depression. Anderson (1998) conducted a meta-analysis of 25 comparative studies on depressed in-patients, and found a slight advantage for tricylics. However, given that the difference was small, one has to agree with Parker (2001) that it is reasonable to offer most patients SSRIs as first-line treatment, but to consider a tricylic only if they fail.

The monoamine oxidase inhibitors (MAOIs) are also no longer widely used, except as second-line choices (Riederer *et al.*, 2004). The problem derives from their side effects, which include serious hypertensive episodes. While these problems occur only in a minority of patients, prevention requires a special diet low in tyramine – a regime not all patients will follow. (More recently developed MAOIs have reversible effects that do not require a special diet.)

6.3 NEWER ANTIDEPRESSANTS

SSRIs were specifically *designed* to treat depression – based on the theory that serotonin transmission is abnormal in patients with low mood. That theory turned out to be dubious. Yet the drugs were a great success.

The first SSRI on the market, fluoxetine, became one of the most widely prescribed drugs of all time. Tolerability was the driving factor behind its popularity. It had fewer side effects and was safer than tricylics.

Even so, SSRIs have problems. One needs to warn patients to endure some unpleasant initial side effects (particularly nausea). A loss of sexual function is all too common, particularly among patients who have reached middle age (Fava and Rankin, 2002). Another problem is that there can be a withdrawal syndrome after stopping the drug, associated with headache, nausea and lethargy (Haddad, 1999), requiring gradual tapering of the dose.

But compared to the precautions required for many drugs that physicians prescribe, such problems were relatively minor. Family doctors, who were never happy with tricyclics, became comfortable enough to use SSRIs fairly routinely.

After fluoxetine, a large number of SSRIs entered the market. The list is now rather long, with the most popular being paroxetine, sertraline, citalopram, (and many other competitors in a crowded field). Yet there is little reason to believe that any of the other SSRIs is consistently better than (or that much different from) fluoxetine. (I will discuss two conflicting studies later that weigh in on that issue.) But for reasons that are not understood, some patients do better on one SSRI than another.

It would help if we knew how SSRIs work. Whatever the mechanism, it does not simply depend on central serotonin activity. Notably, tianeptine, an antidepressant drug used in Europe, is a serotonin reuptake *enhancer* rather than a reuptake inhibitor (DeSimone *et al.*, 1992). One would think such an agent would *make* people depressed. Yet tianeptine has similar effects to SSRIs.

Several non-SSRI antidepressants have been developed. Many are now commonly prescribed, either as first-line or second-line choices. Venlafaxine is the most popular. It was originally marketed as an improvement on SSRIs, and its advertisements emphasized a dual action on 5-HT and NE (i.e., a serotonin-norepinephrine reuptake inhibitor, or SNRI). But there is no evidence that it is superior to an SSRI. Once again, we do not know enough about the relationship between neurotransmitters and depression to make any useful predictions from mechanism to clinical effectiveness.

The manufacturers of venlafaxine made great efforts to convince physicians to use it as a first-line agent. Some studies suggested that remissions of depression might be more frequent than for SSRIs (Thase, Entsuah, and Rudolph, 2001), these industry-sponsored comparative trials have never been independently confirmed. The claim that venlafaxine has fewer sexual side effects has also not been supported by research, while withdrawal problems with this drug are similar (if not worse) as with SSRIs (Haddad, 1999). Moreover, venlafaxine can cause hypertension, and is more dangerous on overdose than SSRIs (Deshauer, 2007). Thus, while it is good to have an alternative, there seems little reason to prefer this drug as a first-line treatment for depression. Even so, venlafaxine continues to be heavily prescribed, and as its patent ran out, the company made it available in extended release form.

Recently, duloxetine has also entered the market as a SNRI, but this agent does not yet have the same depth of research as venlafaxine.

Bupropion is another antidepressant claiming a dual action on 5-HT and NE. It is frequently prescribed for smoking cessation, and has been used to augment other drugs for depression (Thase *et al.*, 2005). While it has been quite successful on the market, there is no reason to prefer it over SSRIs. And as we will see, the evidence does not provide strong support for bupropion as an augmenting agent for depression. Nonetheless, it is common for patients to receive this drug on top of other antidepressants.

Mirtazapine is a tetracyclic that also claims a dual action (Gorman, 1999). This is another drug that has been successful on the market, although the literature does not show any advantages over its competitors (Watanabe *et al.*, 2008). The main point in its favor could be that mirtazapine is highly sedating, helping patients with insomnia.

Buspirone is unrelated chemically to other antidepressants, but it acts as a serotonin agonist. This drug has been used both for depression and for anxiety disorders (Rickels *et al.*, 1991), but it has not had a major impact on the market.

In conclusion, the non-SSRIs offer useful alternatives, but do not supplant them. None have been shown to be more effective than SSRIs (Shelton, 2004) – or for that matter, to tricyclics.

6.4   HOW EFFECTIVE ARE MODERN ANTIDEPRESSANTS?

Antidepressants have provided one of the largest and most lucrative markets in the history of medicine and pharmacology. However, recent research shows that they are not as effective as once thought.

The key to this story is our old friend, the placebo effect. People with depression are "demoralized" (Frank and Frank, 1991), and most are searching for hope. For this reason, many depressed patients are highly open to suggestion. The expectation that one will feel better if one takes a medication is a powerful suggestion. Thus, placebo effects in antidepressant treatment account for 80% of the variance – an even higher percentage than when placebos are used for pain (Kirsch *et al.*, 2008).

In contrast, patients with melancholic depressions cannot easily be reassured. They interpret almost anything in a negative light. That helps to explain why the placebo effect in these cases is very low, as shown by Kirsch *et al.* (2008).

By and large, depressions are the result of gene-environment interactions, and mild or moderate depressions almost always have psychosocial precipitants (Kendler and Prescott 2006). In contrast, melancholic depressions can come "out of the blue," and affect people who have no good reason to be depressed (Parker, 2005; Parker and Manicavasagar, 2005). Thus, the more reasons you have to be depressed, the less likely it is that you will respond to antidepressants.

The size of the placebo effect in the treatment of depression has been seriously underestimated. Its strength only came to light when the results of clinical trials were meta-analyzed *including unpublished trials*. In the past, industry suppressed negative findings for many RCTs (see Chapter 3). That was the reason for establishing new regulations requiring the registration of clinical trials (Laine *et al.*, 2007).

An article in the *New England Journal of Medicine* (Turner *et al.*, 2008) showed that when *unpublished* clinical trials for antidepressants are included in meta-analyses, much less positive results emerge than had been suggested by findings that made it into print. Kirsch *et al.* (2008), using a similar database, conducted a meta-analysis of 47 studies examining the most commonly prescribed SSRIs. The authors showed that when both published and unpublished trials are included, antidepressants were not better than placebo in mild to moderate cases. SSRIs were clearly superior in severe cases, where the placebo response (as one might expect) was quite modest (10% instead of 40–50%).

The strength of the placebo effect in the treatment of depression had previously been underlined in a Cochrane Review (Moncrieff, Wessely, and Hardy, 2004). But the article by Kirsch *et al.* (2008) got more attention in the media. In fact, it created something of a firestorm. Kirsch himself (2009) amusingly describes how "a mild-mannered professor" became an overnight celebrity. The data, reported in almost every major newspaper, raised doubts all over the world as to how useful antidepressants really are.

Some pounced on these results to dismiss antidepressants entirely. Kirsch (2009) himself wrote a book describing their effects as a "myth." Joanna Moncrieff (2008), the first author of a 2004 Cochrane report, also wrote a book arguing that SSRIs are not useful, and that psychosocial methods are greatly superior. Such responses are a vast over-interpretation of findings that should have been considered cautionary, but not in any way debunking. In a later article, Moncrieff and Cohen (2009) were more judicious, suggesting that patients be told that drugs can be prescribed for symptom relief, but that other methods of treatment will probably be needed.

The question of whether antidepressants are truly superior to placebo is a complex problem. Placebo effects in depression have been increasing (Walsh *et al.*, 2002) – possibly because of the impression everyone has that they must be highly effective. Now, with the publicity given to the debunkers, placebo effects may decrease.

The main problem with reaching conclusions derives from the methodology of the clinical trials on which the meta-analyses were based. Almost all were limited by small and not very representative samples. Even more seriously, RCTs are generally too brief (just a few weeks) to have real clinical relevance. It is also possible that placebo effects may wear off with time, while antidepressants may continue to be effective. To find out, we need research that follows depressed patients over longer periods of time.

Some wags have suggested that the most depressing news for patients would be that the drugs they have been taking don't work. But it would be wrong to conclude from meta-analyses that antidepressants are "nothing but placebos." The challenge of these findings should be a stimulus for further research, to identify *which* patients are most likely to respond to drug treatment. For example, a recent meta-analysis (Kaymaz *et al.*, 2008) showed that when depression is recurrent, the advantage of drugs over placebo is greater.

Another line of evidence suggesting that drugs are effective is that patients who have an episode of depression are more likely to relapse if they discontinue their antidepressants (Viguera, Baldessarini, and Friedberg, 1999; Hansen *et al.*, 2008; Kaymaz *et al.*, 2009). Relapse and recurrence are also markers for severity.

Research that puts all major depressions in the same box loses sight of these nuances. Confusing "garden-variety" cases with severe depression only muddies the waters.

In response to the challenge of the Kirsch *et al.* report, major psychiatric journals featured editorials by leading experts in the field (e.g., Thase, 2008; Blier, 2008; Nelson, Thase, and Khan, 2008). Some articles shed doubt on the validity of Kirsch *et al.*'s statistical methods. Others raised questions as to what level of response constitutes clinically significant change or a remission. (Hardly any of the studies in the Kirsch *et al.* meta-analysis measured full remission of depression, either with drug or placebo.) Thus, there is an important difference between short-term remission and sustained recovery.

Thase (2008, p. 487) nicely summarized the limitations of most RCTs on antidepressants: "these studies – which are primarily conducted to obtain regulatory approval, to introduce new medications, or to showcase particular advantages of newer drugs after regulatory approval – form an inadequate basis for an evidence-based medicine assessment of antidepressant effectiveness."

Yet the most searching commentary came from an editorial by Parker (2009), who emphasized the problem in assessing the efficacy of treatment when we have no valid way of diagnosing depression. Parker underlined that antidepressants work best on patients who have the most severe symptoms. Yet researchers rarely conduct RCTs on severely depressed patients. The studies on which most reports are based were conducted on less sick out-patients (or on volunteers recruited by advertisements). Only mild to moderately ill patients will ever sign up for an RCT, while the most severely depressed patients do not. Thus the patients who need drug therapy the most are rarely found in clinical trials. If all RCTs are conducted in samples with milder depressions, it is no wonder that they failed to show much advantage over placebo. That makes it difficult to draw clinical implications, even from meta-analyses.

I believe that critics like Kirsch and Moncrieff have performed an important service for psychiatry. But their dismissal of antidepressants can only be called irresponsible. Based on their own data, they should have concluded that SSRIs (and other antidepressants) are more effective in severe depression, but are much less useful for patients who are either mildly depressed or just unhappy.

Ultimately, it is the current classification system for mood disorders that has misled us. Depression is not a unitary diagnosis, and treatment is not unitary either.

6.5 WHICH ANTIDEPRESSANT?

Physicians have a very large number of antidepressants to choose from. Given the market for these drugs, it is not surprising that efforts have been made to convince them that one or another is particularly advantageous for patients. But does it actually make a difference which one they prescribe?

In a systematic and large-scale meta-analysis, the American College of Physicians (Gartlehner *et al.*, 2008) concluded that it does not. The research group stated (Qaseem *et al.*, 2008, p. 725): "Current evidence does not warrant the choice of one second-generation antidepressant over another on the basis of differences in efficacy and effectiveness." The authors recommended choosing an antidepressant on the basis of side effect profiles and patient preferences.

On the other hand, an equally systematic and large-scale meta-analysis (Cipriani *et al.*, 2009), published at about the same time, came to somewhat different conclusions (p. 746): "Clinically important differences exist between commonly prescribed antidepressants for both efficacy and acceptability in favor of escitalopram and sertraline. Sertraline might be the best choice when starting treatment for moderate to severe major depression in adults because it has the most favorable balance between benefits, acceptability, and acquisition cost."

Who to believe? There was quite a bit of overlap in the data reviewed by both groups. But some of the studies that entered the meta-analyses were funded by industry, further muddying the waters. In the end, their different conclusions depended on how one interprets statistics. If one drug is a few percentage points better than another, is that a clinically significant difference, given the number of patients for whom we prescribe antidepressants? Moreover, can one conclude anything from methods comparing effect sizes in different placebo-controlled RCTs – as opposed to (much rarer) head-to-head comparisons?

If one were to follow the American conclusions, then a choice of antidepressant would depend mostly on which drug one is most familiar with. (That is the advice I usually give when providing consultations to primary care physicians). Other than that, it would be guesswork to make a choice. And, as we will see, if you go on to a second agent when the first fails, it also doesn't seem to make much difference what group your second choice comes from.

If we were to follow the conclusions of Cipriani et al., then we might favor the two drugs found to be most effective. Even so, these differences were not sufficiently large to suggest using either of these drugs on a routine basis. I would not be unhappy if sertraline became the favored choice: this drug is generic, so using it would save everyone a lot of money. On the other hand, escalitopram is still under patent, and patients complain about its price. Physicians always need to think what drugs cost – either for the patient, for the taxpayer, or for insurance companies. By and large, these choices may have to be made on the basis of how well patients tolerate these agents, rather than on dramatic differences in efficacy.

6.6 AUGMENTATION AND SWITCHING: THE STAR*D STUDY

There is now a very large body of research on "treatment-resistant depression." Only about a third of patients remit with a single course of antidepressants, and many patients do not respond, or do not fully respond, to drug treatment of any kind (Moncrieff, 2004; Moncrieff and Kirsch, 2005). But can levels of response be improved with further treatment? This question underlies strategies for the management of treatment-resistant depression, defined as either failure to respond to an antidepressant or a partial response (improvement without remission) (Fava and Davidson, 1996).

If it is seen in two-thirds of all patients after a single course of drug therapy, treatment resistance is hardly a minority phenomenon. And some patients who do not benefit from drugs go on to develop chronic depression (Rubinow, 2004).

Which strategies are most effective to increase the level of response? Standard approaches include: (1) optimizing the dose; (2) switching to another drug; (3) augmenting by adding a second drug.

Psychiatrists are generally good at optimizing doses (and giving drugs for long enough to determine if they are working). However, non-specialists sometimes prescribe too little, and give up too soon. This is a scenario where a consultation can often be helpful.

If these procedures have been properly followed, the main alternatives are augmentation and switching. (Non-pharmacological methods will be considered in Chapter 9.) However, research was needed to determine whether these methods really work.

The large-scale Sequenced Treatment Alternatives to Relieve Depression (STAR*D), a study funded by the National Institute for Mental Health (NIMH), was specifically designed to examine augmentation and switching (Valenstein, 2006). This six-year, $35 million study examined a series of "next best" steps for patients with major depressive disorder who did not benefit from initial treatment. The results have been published in high-impact journals (Rush *et al.*, 2004, 2006a, 2006b; Trivedi *et al.*, 2006a, 2006b; Fava *et al.*, 2004).

Effectiveness studies examine what works in the real world of clinical practice. In this case, the design also included some elements of efficacy research. The trials were divided into four levels, each consisting of RCTs of augmentation and switching (lasting 10–14 weeks) for patients who had not responded at the previous level.

The study was conducted at 41 sites (including both primary and specialized clinics), in which 2876 patients aged 18–75 were recruited. This made the sample fairly clinically representative.

Treatment at Level 1 consisted of citalopram (mean dose of 55 mg). Twenty-eight percent of patients remitted at this stage. Level 2 consisted of RCTs to examine either augmentation or switching. But in an unusual twist, patients were given a choice as to which type of treatment they would prefer, to maximize the "real-world" aspect of the study. The options for switching (chosen by 51% of patients) included sertraline, venlafaxineXR, or bupropionSR. The options for augmentation (chosen by 39% of patients) were buspirone or bupropionSR. Of those who switched, an additional 25% reached remission, although there was no difference among the various alternatives. Of those who chose augmentation, an additional 33% reached remission, again with no difference among the alternatives.

Another option offered to patients was 16 sessions of cognitive therapy. The results showed that remission rates were no better with CBT than with an alternative drug, and they took longer to achieve. But only 25% of subjects accepted randomization to CBT – not really surprising, since they had signed up for a study focusing on drug treatment. For this reason, STAR*D was not a fair test of this well-established alternative to drug therapy. Moreover, the number of sessions offered (16 sessions) was probably insufficient.

At level 3, patients were offered a switch to mirtazapine or nortriptyline, or augmentation to either lithium or thyroid hormone (T3). There was some further value to this switch, in that 20% of those given augmentation responded (thyroid was better tolerated than lithium). Finally, level 4 was offered to all those who were still symptomatic, with a switch to tranylcypromine or mirtazapine plus venlafaxineXR. Another 10% remitted at this final stage.

In the end, two thirds of all patients in the study remitted from depression. This finding seems encouraging, given that only one third responded at the first level. On the other hand, most depressions remit spontaneously with time, and patients who reached levels 3 and 4 had several months to do so. Since this was an effectiveness trial, not an efficacy trial, one cannot say that treatment actually doubled the therapeutic response. In the absence of a placebo control, it is impossible to know whether all outcomes were really drug effects. By the time the study was over, patients had time to recover naturalistically.

Even so, a third of patients still saw no benefit at the end. And the results of augmentation were not that striking. Thus, while the addition of buproprion (a very common strategy in practice) or buspirone yielded statistically significant reductions in HAM-D scores (Trivedi et al., 2006a), the actual differences in response were quite small. One would need to see a larger effect size to justify the routine use of two antidepressants. Moreover, effectiveness studies cannot be as convincing as clinical trials (that should ideally not be industry-sponsored). While some efficacy studies have supported the use of multiple antidepressants (Blier *et al.*, in press), meta-analyses are needed to support this practice.

Fava and Rush (2006, p. 139) came to the following conclusion about augmentation:

> Evidence for these pharmacological approaches rests primarily on open, uncontrolled studies, and there are clearly not enough controlled studies. Clinicians should carefully weigh these different treatment options to increase their patients' chances of achieving and sustaining remission from depression.

Finally, there could be an entirely different explanation for the results seen in the STAR*D study. As suggested by Kirsch (2009), switching and augmentation could have functioned as placebos by raising expectations of improvement in patients. This is a very serious possibility. Again one cannot know the answer in the absence of control groups.

There are several lessons from STAR*D. First, it suggests that patients who fail an initial trial with an antidepressant should be tried on a second one. But contrary to previous clinical wisdom, it did not make a difference whether you switch to another SSRI or choose a completely different group.

Second, when two trials fail, further attempts at switching and augmentation will probably only yield further benefit in a small number of patients. The law of diminishing returns sets in rapidly. Thus the common practice of trying patients on four or five antidepressants in the hope that one will eventually work is not evidence-based medicine.

Third, augmentation is a back-up strategy that should be considered – even if its effects are modest. In the RCT literature, there is fairly good evidence that lithium is the most useful of all augmenters (Bauer and Dopfmer, 1999). But STAR*D showed that patients do not tolerate it easily. The less toxic, but clinically popular, practice of augmenting with bupropion yielded unimpressive results.

STAR*D did not examine the effectiveness of adding a neuroleptic to an antidepressant. This option, discussed in Chapter 5, has better evidence to justify its use in severe depression, and should not be used as a first-line treatment. While some patients may benefit, we need more data to support the use of neuroleptics as augmenters for treatment-resistant cases.

Another limitation of STAR*D is that it did not properly test CBT, either as an alternative to or an addition to drugs. Other evidence for this option will be discussed in Chapter 9. Finally, the researchers never examined the effectiveness of ECT.

STAR*D was a complex study, but it did not shed a strongly positive light on current strategies to manage treatment-resistant depression. In the light of these findings, patients should be informed at the very beginning of treatment that antidepressants may or may not work. Psychiatrists who believe (and convince their patients) that success is just a matter of finding the "right" drug, or mixture of drugs, are raising expectations that cannot be met, and may only succeed in creating a short-lived placebo effect.

6.7   GUIDELINES FOR PRACTICE

One might think that with all the research that has been published on depression, psychiatry had reached a consensus on treatment. That is not so. There is a striking discrepancy between the clinical guidelines published by NICE (Middleton, Shaw, and Feder, 2005) and those published by the American Psychiatric Association (APA, 2002).

The British guidelines do not recommend *any* antidepressant as a routine treatment for mild depression. Instead they advise that drugs be reserved for more serious cases. In contrast, the US guidelines recommend SSRIs as a standard first-line treatment. In my view, the evidence supports British common sense over American enthusiasm.

The crucial issue for practice is how to determine which patients are most likely to benefit from drugs. If depression is not a unitary category of illness, it should not be surprising that antidepressants do not always work.

Patients who are depressed can have other diagnoses. For example, a lowered mood is frequently associated with substance abuse and personality disorders, groups that are less likely to respond to antidepressants (Torrens *et al.*, 2005; Newton-Howes, Tyrer, and Johnson,

2006). If a patient is drinking heavily and taking drugs, substance problems need to be addressed first. If a patient has chronic problems at work and in social relationships, these patterns, depressing in their own right, will need to be addressed in a different way.

Another predictor of a poorer response is chronicity and lack of periods of remission. While patients with recurrent unipolar depression may do well with drugs, those with dysthymia show less consistent improvement (Kocsis, 2003). Moreover, dysthymia, particularly when it has an early onset, is strongly associated with personality disorder (Pepper *et al.*, 1995), conditions in which antidepressants do not yield striking improvements in mood (Paris, 2008c).

In view of the strong placebo response in mild depression, and the uncertain effects of drugs, I consider the NICE guidelines to be right in not recommending the prescription of antidepressants on a first visit. Unlike the APA guidelines, NICE suggests starting with diet, exercise, and a wait-and-see approach. Some patients improve without drugs – particularly after a systematic and empathic evaluation. And if they are not better a week later, little is lost by delay. Once you start a patient on medication, you cannot know whether the improvement you observe represents a placebo response or a therapeutic response. But if a patient does not recover with conservative management, one should certainly try an antidepressant. Even so, we lack the data to identify with precision which patients are most likely to remit with pharmacological therapy.

6.8 ANTIDEPRESSANTS AND SUICIDALITY

There has been a lively controversy about whether SSRI antidepressants increase suicidal behavior. This issue (well-publicized both in the medical community and in the media) led the American FDA to put a "black-box warning" on all antidepressants to warn physicians about their use in patients under the age of 25. (As noted in Chapter 3, this issue was the basis of the controversy about the hiring of David Healy in Toronto.)

The observation that antidepressants can activate depressed patients to the point where they may act on their suicidal ideas is not new; this outcome was well-known with tricyclics (Martinez *et al.*, 2005).

The evidence is somewhat contradictory as to whether SSRIs have a specific effect on suicidality. A review of multiple RCTs suggested that suicide attempts are twice as common when these drugs are prescribed (Fergusson, Doucette, and Glass, 2005). However a second review (Gunnell, Saperia, and Ashby, 2005) found an odds ratio of only 1.5, and a third review (Martinez *et al.*, 2005) found no difference at all. Still another meta-analysis found that the effects varied with age, and were most notable in patients under 25 (Stone *et al.*, 2009).

It must be strongly emphasized that the side effect we are talking about is suicidal *behavior*. None of these studies observed any increase in suicide *completion*. The one study that specifically focused on this outcome (Khan *et al.*, 2003) found completions to be no higher with SSRIs than with placebo.

Thus, SSRIs can make people *feel* more suicidal, and may also lead some patients to make attempts. That does not mean patients are more likely to *commit* suicide after taking these drugs. It is also possible that deaths might occur if patients with severe depression fail to receive treatment. Physicians should be on the watch for increased agitation (which can be associated with suicidality), but should not worry that antidepressants will kill their patients.

I agree with an editorial in BMJ by Cipriani, Barbul, and Geddes (2005), which argued that the benefits of antidepressants outweigh these potential harms. There is no reason to stop prescribing drugs for fear of suicide in an age group. Unfortunately, that is exactly what seems to have happened, especially since the FDAs "black-box warning" implied a particular risk for children and adolescents (Bhatia *et al.*, 2008). Physicians have been frightened away from prescribing SSRIs. There are many problems with these drugs, but suicide is not one of them.

6.9   THE RELUCTANCE TO PRESCRIBE ECT

Thus far we have been talking about drug treatment. But electroconvulsive therapy also has a strong evidence base in melancholic and psychotic depressions (Fink and Taylor, 2007; Shorter and Healy, 2007). ECT, when properly prescribed, yields a more rapid response with fewer side effects than a series of trials with antidepressants. And in such cases, patients are often too sick to wait.

Why is ECT not prescribed more often? There are many explanations, some of which are determined by the media and by the popular prejudice against "shocking people." However another part of the problem comes from the *culture* of psychopharmacology.

Because nobody knows how ECT works, psychiatrists see it as less "scientific" than drugs. It is seen as a blunt instrument that "just happens" to be effective. We like to rationalize our treatments, and when we prescribe drugs, we imagine we are carrying out a fine-grained procedure that changes how neurotransmitters act in the brain. The association with neuroscience is compelling. Unfortunately, this idea is an illusion. But the result is that patients who might have gotten better with ECT often are not receiving it, except as a "last resort."

A complaint often raised about ECT concerns its effect on memory. As documented by a recent review (Fraser, O'Carroll, and Ebmeier, 2008), one can see a loss of autobiographical memory after treatment (although less with unilateral ECT and low voltages). Yet compared to the suffering produced by severe depression, this side effect seems tolerable. Again, there is something about this procedure that makes us less tolerant of side effects than when we are prescribed drugs.

6.10   ANTIDEPRESSANTS AS ANXIOLYTICS

Antidepressants have good evidence for efficacy in both panic and generalized anxiety disorders, as confirmed by meta-analysis (Casacalenda and Boulanger, 1998). Clinical trials have also been conducted in social phobia (van Vliet, den Boer, and Westenberg, 1994), although the boundaries between an anxiety disorder and normal shyness remain unclear (Wakefield *et al.*, 2004).

Antidepressants have long been used for obsessive-compulsive disorder (OCD), and are often given in high doses, even if they rarely produce a full remission (Heyman and Fineberg, 2006). In OCD, highly serotonergic antidepressants (SSRIs and the tricyclic cloimpramine) are more effective; this is one of the few findings in the entire psychopharmacological literature that supports a serotonergic theory of *any* mental disorder – or shows that it makes a difference which antidepressant is prescribed.

Thus antidepressants are as "anxiolytic" as benzodiazepines. The only reason this has not been more obvious is that they act more slowly.

The older drugs, popularly referred to as "benzos," are still very much in use, either by themselves, or as adjuncts to other medication.

These days new anxiolytics are not entering the market, probably because SSRIs are filling the niche. It was not always so. Previously called "minor tranquilizers," anxiolytic drugs had a great impact on psychiatric practice. In the 1950s and 1960s, the trade names of drugs like meprobamate (Miltown) and diazepam (Valium) became household terms that found their way into media articles, books, and even popular songs (Tone, 2008).

We actually know how benzodiazepines work – by increasing the binding of GABA. (This is one of the few examples in which a mechanism of action has been established for a psychiatric drug.) Because they are agonists for the transmitter most involved in inhibitory pathways, benzodiazepines are also potent anticonvulsants.

In psychiatry and in family practice, benzodiazepines are most often used for insomnia (Holbrook *et al.*, 2000), or when an immediate effect (e.g., to control panic attacks) is needed, and/or when antidepressants have not yet taken effect. But benzos have relatively short half-lives, with effects that wear off rapidly with time. They demonstrate marked tolerance, can be addictive, and are cross-tolerant with alcohol and other sedatives (O'Brien, 2005). Fortunately, the problem of addiction emerges only with some patients – as with alcohol, some people can take these drugs for years without increasing the dose (Juergens, 1993).

Benzodiazepines vary in whether they are short, medium, or long-acting, and abuse is most likely with agents that have a rapid action (Woods, Katz, and Winger, 1988). Thus short-acting drugs such as alprazolam may be useful for panic attacks that need to be rapidly aborted. But because these drugs are more likely to produce habituation, long-acting benzos such as clonazepam are now generally preferred. That drug has also long been available as a generic.

Another problem with benzodiazepines concerns their use in the elderly, where they can reduce cognitive function and also be responsible for dangerous falls (Grad, 1997). They should therefore generally be avoided in geriatric practice.

Benzodiazepines continue to be widely prescribed. By 1989, a British survey showed that 7% of the population had taken them within the last year (Taylor, 1989), and there is no reason to believe that the situation has changed in the last two decades. Moreover, patients with major mental illnesses often receive benzos as adjunctive medication (Brunette *et al.*, 2003).

It is a little surprising that drug companies have not come up with a second generation of anxiolytics. In spite of their widespread use, few new drugs of that type have come on the market in recent years. But industry has concentrated on developing new antidepressants, and the market for those drugs has been, up to now, almost limitless.

6.11   ANTIDEPRESSANTS: CLINICAL CONCLUSIONS

I began by saying that antidepressants are overprescribed. Their use has also quadrupled over the past decade (Olfson and Marcus, 2009). Patients may not always like them, if we are to judge by a survey in the US that showed that 43% of patients discontinue them in the first few weeks (Olfson *et al.*, 2006). But one sees many other patients who take these drugs for years.

The problem is not that antidepressants are ineffective, but that we do not know enough about depression to prescribe them in a rational and precise way. I am therefore inclined to approve the conservatism espoused by the NICE guidelines. However, I must acknowledge that there are times when alternatives to drugs are either not available, or no more likely to be successful. In such cases I may recommend a prescription on the grounds that nothing is lost by doing so, and by the chance that some symptoms may at least be reduced. Moreover, the relative innocuousness of drugs like SSRIs encourages us to offer these agents liberally.

This having been said, a great deal of time, effort, and money is lost trying to find the right cocktail for every depressed patient. There is still no substitute for understanding the life problems of patients. Depression is not always a disease.

CHAPTER 7

Prescribing for Children and Adolescents

Children and adolescents are a special population. They may not suffer from the same mental disorders as adults. They also may not respond to the same drugs, or need the same doses of agents that are effective for similar symptoms in adults. Moreover, there has long been a dearth of clinical trials of drugs in child populations, although, as we will see, this situation is improving.

Another way that children are special is that they are not capable of providing informed consent. Thus pharmacological management of disorders in childhood always depends on an alliance with the family. But parents may be even more concerned about their children than they are for themselves. For this reason, and because we all feel a special responsibility to our youngest patients, there is sometimes a strong pressure to "do something" rapidly with drugs, even when a more patient and cautious approach is indicated. Not every child with symptoms needs pharmacological treatment, and when they do, the general rule should be "start low, go slow."

7.1 STIMULANTS

Stimulants are among the most extensively studied of all psychiatric drugs. A vast literature (Barkley, 2006) supports the efficacy of methylphenidate for attention deficit hyperactivity disorder (ADHD). Yet not every case of ADHD responds to this agent (or its long-acting variants). While other stimulants have been tried (d-amphetamine, modafanil), as well as non-stimulants (atomoxetine, tricyclic antidepressants, buproprion, guanfacine), about 30% of children with ADHD are resistant to any drug (Owens, Hinshaw, and Arnold, 2003; Cumyn *et al.*, 2007). And while longer-acting stimulants have been widely used, there is little evidence that they produce a more robust response (Faraone and Glatt, 2009).

What is the explanation? As we have seen, drugs often yield different responses in different individuals. This is a problem that runs through all of psychiatry, not to speak of the rest of medicine. But there is another problem, one that we have already seen in depression: ADHD is a heterogeneous diagnosis. Deficits in attention and increases in activity are a syndrome with many causes, not a well-defined disease category.

We do not yet know how to define the boundaries of ADHD with any degree of precision. Like other mental disorders, the diagnosis depends entirely on signs and symptoms, not on a blood test or a brain scan. Even though biological tests in medicine are not always definitive, they would provide a framework that is intrinsically more reliable than observation alone.

Moreover, the category of ADHD is part of a larger spectrum of disruptive behavior disorders, all of which overlap greatly (Jensen, Martin, and Cantwell, 1997). In practice, it is often "comorbid" diagnoses (usually conduct disorder) that bring children with ADHD to clinical attention (Schachar and Tannock, 2002).

While ADHD is sometimes identified using neuropsychological testing, such results are non-specific, and not really necessary for diagnosis. One of the most common measures is the Continuous Performance Test (CPT) – a deliberately boring task designed to measure sustained attention – on which patients with ADHD show abnormal results. However while the CPT separates cases from normal controls, it fails to differentiate ADHD from other disruptive behavioral disorders (McGee *et al.*, 2000).

A "rough and ready" measure in frequent use for identifying ADHD is the Conners' Rating Scales–Revised (Kollins *et al.*, 2006). This is a checklist that parents and teachers can fill out, describing the clinical features of ADHD. But since the items differ little from DSM-IV-TR criteria, the Conners is in no way an independent "gold standard" for diagnosis.

Another twist is that ADHD describes more than one syndrome. DSM-IV-TR describes three subtypes – hyperactive, inattentive, and mixed. The hyperactive type corresponds most closely to the original diagnostic construct of attention deficit disorder that stimulants were intended to treat. The inattentive type is less well defined (Morgan *et al.*, 1996), and response to stimulants in such cases is much less consistent (Carlson and Mann, 2000). It remains to be seen as to whether the expansion of ADHD will prove to have been based in solid science. Moreover, there are other diagnoses in which children can be inattentive – other externalizing conditions (such as conduct disorder and oppositional defiant disorder), as well as internalizing disorders (such as anxiety and depression).

Diagnosis of childhood disorders of any kind tends to be more problematic than in adults. Comorbidity is extremely common, and boundaries for each category fuzzy. Even if children meet criteria for three or four disorders, that does not mean they have more than one disease. Rather, multiple diagnoses reflect the overlapping criteria we use to make diagnoses. Many of these conditions (conduct disorder, ADHD) have separate clinical and research literatures, but may be describing some of the same phenomena in different theoretical frameworks.

To deal with this problem, psychological symptoms in childhood can be described using two broad dimensional constructs: *externalizing* and *internalizing* (Achenbach and McConaughy, 1997). Even in adulthood, most DSM-IV defined disorders can also be factor analyzed into these dimensions (Krueger, 1999). While such broad spectra are not diagnoses, they are useful in that they take into account the commonalities between existing categories, which are not based in unique pathological processes.

ADHD is a good example of an externalizing disorder. It may not be a specific medical diagnosis with a specific treatment. Yet labeling the syndrome is useful if it helps to guide choice of treatment, specifically a group that responds predictably to stimulants.

One sees classical cases of ADHD that do not present these diagnostic problems. Even then, there can be more than one option for treatment. While most US physicians would immediately choose stimulants, the NICE guidelines (2008) take a different view. As in depression (NICE, 2007), British psychiatrists prefer conservative management: watchful waiting and increasing environmental structure first, with a move to medication only when that strategy fails. (Once again, there seems to be a consistent cultural difference between American activism and British caution.)

If conservative management does not reduce the disability associated with ADHD, then stimulants are the best documented alternative. In a large multi-centered trial in which children were offered methylphenidate with or without multimodal psychosocial interventions, the drug was *by far* the most effective choice (Hechtman *et al.*, 2004). Thus psychological interventions do not have as strong an evidence base as stimulants. But comorbidity can influence the course of treatment (Pelham and Fabian, 2008). Also, Owens, Hinshaw, and Arnold (2003) noted that ADHD patients with conduct disorder are more likely to benefit from psychological interventions. The larger question is whether stimulants are mainly of benefit to those with more severe and more classical symptoms (Pelham and Fabian, 2008).

Another limitation of clinical trials is that, as we have seen, samples may not be representative of real world populations. Children who are already in specialized care may need different management from those who are seen in community settings. The NICE guidelines take into account the mild cases that meet ADHD criteria, but may not need stimulants.

Can ADHD, either in children or adults, be diagnosed by a specific therapeutic response to stimulants? Classically, it has been thought that hyperactivity shows a paradoxical response, in that children with this symptom become calmer (rather than excited) by a stimulant. However, the effects of stimulants on attention are less specific. As has been known for over three decades, *everyone* has improved attention when taking stimulants (Rapoport *et al.*, 1978). Thus there is no precise way to distinguish ADHD based on therapeutic response.

The presence of comorbidity also influences the response to stimulants. Drugs are less effective when conduct disorder is severe (Earle and Mezzacappa, 2002; Schachar and Tannock, 2002; Owens, Hinshaw, and Arnold, 2003).

Finally, ADHD has a social dimension. In childhood, the syndrome is, at least in part, an artifact of modern educational policy (Barkley, 2006). In previous generations, children who could not tolerate sitting still in a classroom left school early and went to work. That option is no longer permitted in our society. Even in adulthood, there is a difference between the demands of a desk job (which requires a particular type of sustained attention) and traditional occupations that primarily involve physical labor.

In summary, the most characteristic cases of ADHD respond to stimulants. Boundary cases and patients with significant comorbidity may not. This is the same scenario we have seen unfolding for all the major groups of drugs used in psychiatry. And that is why pharmacological treatments can never be prescribed in a routine way.

Children with ADHD do not always improve with maturity, and some continue to require stimulant therapy in adulthood – usually for symptoms of inattention (Weiss and Hechtman, 1992. In many ways, some symptoms are likely to remain present, even if they are subclinical. Even so, adult ADHD is a problematic diagnosis. One should not conclude that inattentiveness is usually a symptom of ADHD. To meet criteria for the adult type, DSM-IV-TR requires that ADHD symptoms begin prior to age 7. While this cutoff could be arbitrary (and DSM-V might change it), the important step of documenting a childhood history is often omitted. Moreover, information about childhood requires independent confirmation. Retrospectively, people tend to remember the past in terms of the present. Clinicians do not always have access to report cards from kindergarten. But they should make a serious effort to find out if symptoms were present from an early age.

I see many patients in adult psychiatry asking if they "have ADHD." The media have encouraged this trend by publicizing the idea that cases are being missed, and that a simple prescription can change a life. Actually, most adult patients with problems in inattention suffer from anxiety, mood, or personality disorders. The symptoms of ADHD in adulthood are at least as non-specific as they are in children.

In adulthood, ADHD tends to be highly comorbid with many other diagnoses (Kessler *et al.*, 2006). About half have substance abuse, personality disorders, or both (Cumyn, Hechtman, and French, 2009). These are not the kind of patients that can be expected to have a dramatic response to stimulants.

In summary, adult ADHD exists, but this is a diagnostic problem that sometimes threatens to be a fad. One cannot even be sure that patients who seem to respond to stimulants have the disorder, given their effects on normal people and the possibility of placebo responses. Biological markers to establish the boundaries of this diagnosis are sorely needed.

7.2   ANTIDEPRESSANTS IN CHILDREN

Several decades ago, psychiatrists accepted that depression can occur before puberty. Depressed children develop very similar symptoms to adults, even if suicidal thoughts are rare (Ryan *et al.*, 1987). But treatment options for children are more complicated. Drugs do not work in the same way at all ages.

When prescribing for younger patients, neurodevelopment has to be taken into account, since drugs affect the growing brain. Neurons grow rapidly and establish new synapses during childhood, and most are then pruned after puberty (Neville and Bavelier, 2000). Many mental disorders begin at puberty, when there is a major reorganization of neural pathways, and when there are large-scale changes in endocrine activity.

That may be the reason why drugs can have very different effects in pre-pubertal children and in adolescents. By and large, adolescents are more like adults than school-aged children.

The literature has been confusing on this point. Thus when a review of antidepressants in pediatric populations (Cheung, Emslie, and Mayes, 2006) uses the word "children" in its title – and then focuses almost entirely on research on adolescents – readers can be misled.

This issue is important for the controversy as to whether antidepressants work the same way in pediatric populations as in adults. Jureidini *et al.* (2004) reviewed the literature and concluded that efficacy in all patients under age 18 is unproven. In contrast, Tsapakis, Soldani, and Baldessarini (2008) and Kutcher (1997) presented evidence for their usefulness in adolescents, while conceding that data in pre-pubertal populations is slim. Bridge *et al.* (2007) conducted a meta-analysis that supported efficacy for antidepressants in adolescents, but when children under the age of 12 were examined separately, most antidepressants were no better than placebo.

Thus antidepressant treatment for major depression in adolescence is not, in principle, different than in adults. But as noted by Raz (2006), the strength of placebo effects has to be taken into account. This is of course the same problem that we have in assessing the efficacy of SSRIs in adults. The Treatment of Adolescents for Depression project (The TADS Team, 2007) conducted effectiveness trials suggesting that SSRIs are useful, although results were better when cognitive behavioral therapy was added. (The advantage of combination therapy at any age will be discussed in Chapter 9). The presence of comorbid diagnoses such as anxiety disorders may also influence the choice of treatment.

There are practical problems that make the assessment and treatment of depression in adolescence difficult. First, normal adolescents have mood swings, probably related to the profound hormonal changes that take place after puberty. Second, substance abuse, which often begins at puberty, can complicate treatment, in that the prescription of antidepressants is much less likely to be effective. Third, it is more difficult to establish an alliance with adolescents, who are less likely to be compliant with drugs. Fourth, one sees quite a bit of diagnostic instability at this stage.

7.3   SUICIDALITY IN ADOLESCENCE

Although there has been wide publicity in the media about the risk of adolescent suicide, completed suicide before the age of 18 remains rare (Pelkonen and Matunnen, 2003). That is not say that completion never happens, or that suicide in an adolescent is not a tragedy if it does occur. But the most prevalent phenomena at this age are not completed suicides, but suicidal thoughts, suicidal attempts, and self-harm. As shown by prospectively followed community samples (Brezo *et al.*, 2007), suicidal thoughts are even more ubiquitous among adolescents than major depression.

In adults, about 15–20% of the population will experience suicidal thoughts at some time (Kessler *et al.*, 2005a). Yet since the rate of completed suicide in the general population is only 0.001%, the presence of suicidal ideas is not useful as a predictor. The principle applies equally to adolescents, who even more rarely kill themselves (prior to age 18 or 19).

Adolescence is the time when suicide attempts, mainly by overdose, begin to occur, and these behaviors are more frequent in girls (Pelkonen and Matunnen, 2003). Psychiatrists have been taught to be alarmed and vigilant about *any* patient who reports suicidal thoughts. But since doing so results in many false positives, high vigilance may create more problems than advantages in practice (Paris, 2006).

The same principles apply to suicide attempts. In longitudinal follow-up studies of adults, Hawton *et al.* (2005) showed that attempts are associated with a completion rate of only 1–2%. Suicidal behaviors should always be a cause for clinical concern, since they reflect distress levels. But an adolescent who takes an overdose is not necessarily at risk of losing their life.

The question of whether SSRI antidepressants can increase suicidality in adults was discussed in Chapter 6. There is no evidence that the problem is any different in adolescents. Thoughts and attempts can become more frequent when adolescents receive antidepressants, but the evidence supports a relationship with suicidal *behaviors*, not with completed suicide (Gibbons, Brown, and Hur, 2007). Moreover, if treatment is successful, as the TADS study suggests it can often be, then it should be worth accepting temporary increases in suicidality in a minority of cases.

7.4 PEDIATRIC BIPOLAR DISORDER

Since the time of Kraepelin (1921), it has been generally accepted that manic symptoms do not develop any earlier than adolescence. The NICE (2009) guidelines for bipolar treatment state that while the disorder can begin before puberty, that is a rare event. But this conclusion has been questioned, and the idea that mania can begin in childhood, and is actually common before puberty, has become influential (Wozniak, 2005; Faedda *et al.*, 2004).

The hypothesis is that affective and behavioral symptoms in childhood are often manifestations of bipolarity. These patterns are associated with a broad emotional dysregulation that tends to persist over time (Geller *et al.*, 2008; Birmaher *et al.*, 2009). Thus, children formerly diagnosed as having ADHD or CD would be seen as having an early form of bipolar disorder.

There is no controversy about the observation that bipolar disorder can begin after puberty. But pre-pubertal children do not have manic or hypomanic episodes. One can only speak of bipolarity if the construct is broadened to include affective dysregulation, irritability, and behavioral symptoms.

In Chapter 5, the concept of a bipolar spectrum was questioned because it is entirely based on phenomenological resemblance. There is no evidence from genetics, neurobiology, or treatment response to show that what is being called pediatric bipolar disorder has anything in common with classical bipolarity. In a recent prospective study of the children of bipolar parents (Duffy *et al.*, 2009), mood disorder episodes (mostly depression) started only after puberty, and no features of bipolarity were observed in the cohort prior to that stage.

Actually, all the symptoms putatively considered to be "bipolar," particularly irritability and impulsivity, are commonly found in children in community studies (Duffy, 2007). These are also the most frequent problems seen in children referred to psychiatrists. When you read descriptions of these patients (Geller *et al.*, 2008), it is clear that these are troubled children, but with unstable mood rather than manic episodes. Geller's group found they were highly comorbid for disruptive behavioral disorders (conduct disorder, oppositional defiant disorder, and ADHD). That is how children with this clinical picture were traditionally diagnosed.

The category of conduct disorder (CD) has a large literature. Almost half a century ago, a long-term follow-up of children showed that psychopathy in adulthood (now called antisocial personality disorder) – is *always* preceded by conduct disorder (Robins, 1966). (In one of the rare cases in which research directly influenced DSM criteria, a diagnosis of antisocial personality cannot be made unless CD has been present before age 15.) But not every case of CD goes on to adult psychopathy, and some develop anxious or depressive symptoms in adulthood; an antisocial outcome is most likely in severe CD (Zoccolillo *et al.*, 1992; Caspi *et al.*, 1996). Tellingly, *none* of the many follow-up studies of CD has ever found bipolar disorder developing in adulthood.

While a diagnosis of CD might better account for symptoms called "bipolar," the construct, like so many other diagnoses in psychiatry is a heterogeneous grab-bag. One only needs 3 out of 15 possible criteria to receive it – children with the same diagnosis may not share any clinical features at all, and CD might eventually be disassembled into smaller pieces.

There is no drug specific for conduct disorder, and available treatment involves costly (albeit effective) behavioral training (Kazdin, 2005). But the temptation to call these problems bipolarity reflects the wish for an easier pharmacological solution.

In the same way, many "bipolar" symptoms are consistent with ADHD. We have data from long-term studies following these children into adulthood (Weiss and Hechtman, 1993; Manuzza and Klein, 2000). This research shows that while some cases remit with time, these children have an increased risk for developing antisocial personality disorder and substance use in adulthood. Once again, *none* of these studies has described an evolution of ADHD into bipolar disorder.

Could there still be a sub-group of cases with behavior disorders that are bipolar variants? The presence of grandiose thinking has been used to distinguish such cases (Geller *et al.*, 2008). But grandiosity in adults with bipolar disorder is associated with delusions and delusional trends. What one sees in a behaviorally disturbed child is simple boastfulness. This is hardly the same phenomenon – except for those who see bipolarity everywhere.

Is there any follow-up data on cases diagnosed as bipolar in childhood that might tell us whether classical bipolarity is an outcome in adulthood? Let us return to the report by Geller *et al.* (2008). One hundred and fifteen cases were followed for eight years, from a mean baseline of 11 years to age 19. The authors reported that their cohort had a 73% rate of relapse of bipolar symptoms. However none of their subjects actually developed mania or hypomania, as classically defined. Instead, about half of the subjects continued to score on a specially designed interview devised to measure "softer" signs of bipolarity that had been described at baseline. These consisted of mood swings, grandiose behaviors, a decreased need for sleep, racing thoughts, and hypersexuality. While these features showed continuity over time, they are also consistent with other diagnoses. In fact, most of these subjects also met criteria for a diagnosis of ADHD and/or oppositional defiant disorder.

Similar findings were reported in another four-year follow-up study of children diagnosed as bipolar (Birmaher *et al.*, 2009). In essence, these reports beg the question as to whether or not the children under study *ever* had a bipolar disorder. Unlike adult cases, these children did not show a dramatic change in mood from baseline, but chronic affective instability. Moreover, most symptoms were behavioral rather than affective, again pointing to a disruptive behavior disorder. Brotman *et al.* (2006) have used the term *severe mood dysregulation* (SMD) – as opposed to bipolar disorder – to describe such cases, and find that these children go on to develop depression, not mania, later in life.

Epidemiological data could shed light on this issue. Yet large-scale studies using *current* diagnostic practices have not identified cases of bipolar disorder before puberty (Duffy, 2006). As noted in Chapter 5, studies of adults only find such cases when they use "soft" signs of bipolarity (Merikangas *et al.*, 2007). Nor has it been shown that the first-degree relatives of putatively bipolar children have bipolar disorders (as classically defined), or that these cases share any biological markers with adult patients who develop bipolar-I or bipolar-II. Finally, children with a bipolar parent, who might be expected to be at particular risk, are generally more likely to develop psychopathology, including bipolar disorders, but there is no evidence that symptoms start in childhood (Singh *et al.*, 2007).

In summary, the existence of bipolar disorder prior to puberty is not proven, nor has continuity with the adult form been demonstrated. While bipolar disorders are both heritable and frequent in the population, like so many other mental disorders (e.g., schizophrenia, and substance abuse) their onset is usually in adolescence. But this controversy is difficult to resolve on the basis of phenomenology alone. As with all diagnoses in psychiatry, the absence of biological markers makes it difficult to establish boundaries between one syndrome and another.

Nonetheless, if it could be shown that cases of pediatric bipolar disorder respond to the same treatments as adult forms, pharmacological dissection might provide some support for the concept. Some studies suggest that mood stabilizers and antipsychotics reduce symptoms in these children (Kowatch *et al.*, 2005), but what one usually sees is clinical improvement on a symptom scale, without the remission in the treatment of adult cases, and there have been no long-term follow-ups. The therapeutic effects that are seen could also be due to non-specific sedation.

In view of all these uncertainties, one must ask whether the benefits of drug treatment in children with behavioral disorders outweigh the risks. Long-term treatment with mood stabilizers and antipsychotics in children is not without consequences. There can be rapid and massive weight gain, which the combination of mood stabilizers and atypical neuroleptics is particularly likely to cause (Correll and Leucht, 2007). It is also possible that children who take atypical neuroleptics for years could develop tardive dyskinesia. Finally, one even hears of psychiatrists treating pre-school children with these drugs (when behavioral problems are seen as bipolar).

In this light, the practice of prescribing mood stabilizers and atypical neuroleptics to pre-pubertal children could only be justified if the diagnosis of pediatric bipolar disorder at this age is valid, and if it can be shown that the sequelae of *not* treating these children carries a greater cost. At this point, the burden of proof lies with those who support the concept, and not with those who, like myself, doubt its validity.

7.5   A CAUTIOUS VIEW OF PSYCHOPHARMACOLOGY IN CHILDHOOD

Behavioral disorders of childhood are a serious problem: they can disrupt the lives of children and their parents. It should therefore not be surprising that psychiatrists want to believe in a pharmacological solution or that parents, at their wit's end, are willing to go along with these regimes. However, the long-term effects of aggressive pharmacotherapy in children are not known. If a child has ADHD, we can at least rest assured that we have decades of data to rely on, but the long-term effects of aggressive pharmacotherapy in children with other disorders are not known. We need more research on this and also on non-pharmacological alternatives, such as parent training, although a meta-analysis of this literature (Lundahl , Risser, and Lovejoy, 2006) suggested that effects are small (and not always stable).

As a general principle, the pharmacological treatment of children should be carried out with extra caution. We should be particularly concerned about prescribing atypical neuroleptics to children; recent surveys show that this practice is increasing dramatically (Crystal *et al.*, 2009). And the concept of a bipolar child who is seen as requiring these agents has to be viewed with concern.

Without strong scientific evidence behind it, aggressive pharmacological treatment in children can only be described as prescribing in the dark. This would not be the first time in history that, with the best intentions, psychiatrists do real harm to their youngest patients. On the one hand, the wish to get behavioral problems under control rapidly is understandable, from the point of view of both the child and the parents (who sometimes feel rather desperate). There may also be a fear that if nothing is done, permanent damage may ensue, but these pressures should not lead to over-treatment. At all ages, drug therapy needs to be cautious, prudent, and watchful.

CHAPTER 8

Polypharmacy

8.1 MEDICINE AND MINIMALISM

Other things being equal, medicine should be practiced with a *minimalist* perspective. Every treatment should be introduced with caution and carefully monitored. Interventions should be calibrated to the minimum level at which results can still be expected. The possibility that patients can get better without treatment should always be entertained. It would be better if psychopharmacology adopted the motto that "less is more."

The climate of psychiatric practice favors drugs – and multiple drugs – particularly when a first (or subsequent) agent fails. But there is a cost to this approach. Polypharmacy, prescribing multiple agents for multiple symptoms, means that patients will suffer from multiple side effects. I am not talking about the use of two drugs, for which, as we have seen, there are evidence-based indications. I am discussing a practice in which patients receive four, five, or even more agents for the same condition.

Polypharmacy is not unique to psychiatry, or to the present era of drug treatment. Over a hundred years ago, William Osler (1898) criticized his colleagues for treating patients with "shotgun" methods, giving drugs to manage each symptom separately and focusing on symptoms rather than on a disease process. Osler's comments still apply to the practice of medicine.

The Use and Misuse of Psychiatric Drugs: An Evidence-Based Critique   by Joel Paris
© 2010 John Wiley & Sons, Ltd

8.2   WHY POLYPHARMACY HAPPENS

Polypharmacy results from a combination of thoughtlessness and a misguided wish to help patients. Some politicians have criticized a tendency to mindlessly "throw money at problems." In medicine, we throw drugs at symptoms. And it is always easier to start a drug than to stop one. In recent years, as shown by as recent survey of psychiatrists in the USA (Mojtabai and Olfson, 2010), the frequency of multiple prescriptions is increasing. No doubt this reflects the fact that prescribing practices have become looser, and as the popularity of the idea that augmentation is a necessary procedure.

One of the ironies of contemporary practice is that the more specialized the physician, the more likely it is that multiple drugs will be prescribed. Today most family doctors are comfortable about offering antidepressants and/or anxiolytics. But they are hesitant to take on patients who, after being treated by psychiatrists, have been on four or five drugs for years. Who can blame them? After all, the expert must have had a reason for prescribing so many agents.

Behind polypharmacy lies one of the driving ideas in contemporary psychiatry: the myth of the "expert consultant." Experts in psychopharmacology, when consulted, tend not to say the medication is doing as much as can be expected, and other modalities of treatment should be considered. Instead, they are likely to favor aggressive treatment with multiple drugs. (The use of the word "aggressive" as a positive rather than as a negative descriptor of this approach already provides cause for concern.)

The armamentarium of the modern expert depends on strategies of augmentation (or switching). Yet, as we have seen in Chapter 6, while this approach sometimes works (and should certainly be considered in treatment-resistant cases), it often fails. But if the strategy does not help the patient, full rethinking of the plan may not ensue. Any further consultations are almost guaranteed to suggest another new drug, an additional drug, or both.

Consumers of treatment have also come to believe that there are effective cocktails that only experts know how to mix. For this reason, the power and charisma of the expert can be more important than the recommended treatment. For all these reasons, placebo effects are particularly likely to be associated with polypharmacy. And like all placebo effects, they may not last for long.

8.3 HOW POLYPHARMACY HAPPENS

In a community study, Patten and Beck (2004) found that 9% of all patients with mental disorders are receiving polypharmacy. That number may be on the low side. Patients with mild depressions seen in primary care may only be given one drug (usually an SSRI, possibly augmented with a benzo for insomnia). The survey did not examine specialty clinics separately, and that is probably the place where polypharmacy is most common. The sickest and most chronic patients with the most complex and intractable problems are the ones who end up on multiple drugs.

This observation gives us a clue as to what the practice of polypharmacy is really about. It is an attempt to deal with treatment-resistance. When one drug does not work, a second is added. When two drugs do not work, a third is added. A common pattern is for patients to end up receiving one drug from each of the major groups (antipsychotics, antidepressants, mood stabilizers, and anxiolytics). This sequence can develop in the treatment of many different conditions, including schizophrenia, depression, bipolar disorder, and personality disorders.

Schizophrenia presents a challenge. One survey found that it is not uncommon for psychotic in-patients to be on more than one neuroleptic (Thompson et al., 2008) – a doubtful practice that has never been evaluated in research. Moreover, when chronically psychotic patients are depressed, they may be prescribed an antidepressant (or a mood stabilizer). A meta-analysis found that this practice is based on very weak evidence (Whitehead et al., 2003). While practitioners often feel the need to do *something* for these patients, why add to the side effect burden?

As we have seen, many depressed patients (and not only those with psychosis or melancholia) are now receiving antipsychotics. There is little evidence for prescribing these agents routinely, or to assume that they are likely to be consistently effective as augmenters. In mild to moderate depression, there is no data to support their use for anything more than insomnia (which can, in any case, be treated in other ways). It is also common for depressed patients to receive mood stabilizers. But while lithium can be helpful in some treatment-resistant depressions, there is no evidence base for its routine use (or the use of anticonvulsant drugs) for chronically depressed patients. Nor is there strong evidence for the use of a second antidepressant in any but the most severe and treatment-resistant cases.

Bipolar patients are particularly likely to receive more than one drug. At one time, monotherapy with mood stabilizers was considered standard. Today, dual therapy (in which antipsychotics are routinely prescribed from the beginning) has become common. As recommended in a recent review (Ketter, 2009), it is usually worth waiting to see if monotherapy works by itself. Another peculiar twist I have observed is the use of multiple mood stabilizers, a practice that has never been empirically tested.

Polypharmacy is common in patients with complex problems such as personality disorders and substance abuse (Ghaemi, 2002). For example, borderline personality disorder, a category with a wide range of symptoms, is notably difficult to treat (Paris, 2008b). For this reason it is not surprising that so many of these patients are on four or five drugs (Zanarini *et al.*, 2001). Yet the evidence base for using any drug in this population is slim (Binks *et al.*, 2006; Paris, 2008c).

When one prescribes one drug from each major group (antipsychotics, mood stabilizers, antidepressants, anxiolytics), the total will be four, but sometimes one sees even more agents prescribed due to doubling up on one of these classes. If this is "aggressive" psychopharmacology, then most of our patients would be better off with a kinder and gentler approach.

8.4 CRITERIA FOR A RATIONAL POLYPHARMACY

Preskorn and Lacey (2007) published a useful and comprehensive review of polypharmacy in psychiatry. Their overall conclusion (p. 104) was: "Although there is an extensive literature on copharmacy, the quality of the reports varies widely. Many are single or multiple case reports without any controls. Some are controlled but may not be double-blind. The few that are properly controlled are typically underpowered and not of sufficient duration to convincingly establish the efficacy, safety, and tolerability of the copharmacy over monodrug therapy."

On the other hand, Ghaemi (2002), author of one of the few book-length treatments of the subject, offers a guarded defense of polypharmacy, arguing that complex pathology may require complex treatment. Even so, he acknowledges that evidence for the practice is usually not present. In fact, there has been surprisingly little research on drug combinations.

The argument made by Ghaemi (2002) is that since mental disorders affect many neurotransmitters, single drugs are likely to be insufficient. Yet, as we have seen, mental illness is not well explained by any neurotransmitter theory. Nor is there any basis for a theory that explains drug effects by their effects on transmitters. As Healy (2009) rightly points out, every drug we use is a cocktail that affects multiple systems. Drugs are not specific to any category of mental illness, but have overlapping effects on many symptoms.

Preskorn and Lacey (2007) proposed a set of 12 criteria for a rational polypharmacy:

1. Knowledge that the combination has a positive effect on the pathophysiology or pathoetiology of the disorder.
2. Convincing evidence that the combination is more effective, including more cost-effective, than monodrug therapy.
3. The combination therapy should not pose significantly greater safety or tolerability risks than monotherapy.
4. The drugs should not interact both pharmacokinetically and pharmacodynamically.
5. Drugs have mechanisms of action that are likely to interact in a way that augments response.
6. Each drug should have only one mechanism of action.
7. Drugs should not have a broad-acting mechanism of action.
8. Drugs should not have the same mechanism of action.
9. Drugs should not have opposing mechanisms of action.
10. Each drug should have simple metabolism.
11. Each drug should have an intermediate half-life.
12. Each drug should have linear pharmacokinetics.

A quick glance at this list should be sufficient to confirm the non-rational nature of polypharmacy. The first criterion should be fairly basic – but we do not know how any of the drugs we use affect etiological and pathogenetic pathways.

As for the second criterion, few direct comparisons of polypharmacy to monotherapy have been carried out, and there are only a few clinical situations in which drug combinations have been shown to be superior. But combining two drugs on the basis of research is quite different from throwing "everything in the book" at the symptoms of complex disorders.

As for the risks associated with polypharmacy, one can only say that they badly need to be researched. With cumulative side effects, safety and tolerability can be real issues.

All the other criteria listed by Preskorn and Lacey concern mechanisms: that is, do two drugs overlap in their action on the brain? In most cases they do. Antidepressants, mood stabilizers, and neuroleptics in particular, all are known to have effects on multiple monoamine systems, not to speak of actions on other major neurotransmitters. And whether these effects have anything to do with the efficacy of drugs remains to be determined. In fact, hardly any of the polypharmacy in current practice comes even close to meeting scientific standards.

8.5   WALKING DOWN THE PRIMROSE PATH

Psychiatrists treat patients with chronic illnesses, many of whom either remain disabled or never fully recover. We want to help our patients by exploring every possible avenue of intervention. Prescribing multiple drugs has much the same motivation as wanting to try "the latest thing" being promoted by industry. We are reluctant to deny patients any chance for remission, even if the odds are against us.

The real reasons behind the use of drug cocktails reflect faulty clinical thinking. Polypharmacy is a response to "treatment resistance," that is, situations when drugs fail to produce remission. But even if initial treatment fails, practitioners may be reluctant to stop any drugs already prescribed, due to fear of relapse. That is how practice walks down the primrose path to polypharmacy.

Treatment-resistance should really not be surprising, considering that we are treating disorders we do not really understand. Prescribing more and more drugs is not necessarily a logical response to that problem. But some psychiatrists know no other way of managing mental illness. Once again, if you only have a hammer, everything looks like a nail. Polypharmacy is a way of hammering away, even when the nail is the wrong size, or when there is no nail at all.

Finally, polypharmacy is driven by a narrow view of disease. If mental disorders are purely biological, then one might think that a purely biological treatment should be effective. As Chapter 9 will demonstrate, the data show that many patients need non-pharmacological treatments, which by and large, they are not being offered.

We need to be more philosophical about our limitations as healers. Many of the chronic illnesses psychiatrists treat do not fully respond to any form of treatment. A mature clinician comes to accept this, and work within the realm of the possible.

One of tragedies of polypharmacy is that patients themselves come to believe in it. Their very identity becomes entangled with how many medications they need. Many have special containers to keep track of every drug they take. Some endlessly seek a magic cocktail that will put an end to their suffering.

When psychiatrists practice on the basis of the same belief, each visit consists of "adjusting" medications – either changing doses or adding something new. Patients who have had a bad week are almost guaranteed an adjustment. There is no evidence that adjusting medication every time a patient is feeling worse constitutes good medicine. At best, this is a practice that produces powerful placebo effects. Over time, medication adjustments become the currency of connection with the physician. Many of our patients are lonely, and are happy to have regular appointments in which their medications are "fussed over." When I consult on a case, I have often found it difficult to convince patients that they do not need all the drugs they have been given by previous physicians.

I am also old enough to remember when another (but very different) magic expert dominated the practice of psychiatry. Forty years ago, practitioners and patients believed that senior psychoanalysts had a deep understanding of the psyche that allowed them to treat almost any symptom successfully (Paris, 2005). In many ways, psychopharmacology has fallen into the very same trap. But at least the main harm that psychoanalysts did was to waste their patients' time and money. Drugs may produce more lasting problems.

While there are clinical situations in which patients require more than one medication, but the indications are narrow. Moreover, the prescription of multiple drugs should never be taken lightly. In most cases, it is better to start with a single agent and observe the response. If there is no improvement within a reasonable time, one can then choose to augment or switch. Yet all too often, new drugs are added and none is ever subtracted. Again, no one has ever studied the effects of three agents (or more) on patients with mental disorders.

In summary, polypharmacy, while based on good intentions, tends to do more harm than good. As Samuel Johnson once said of second marriages, prescribing multiple drugs reflects the triumph of hope over experience.

Perspectives

CHAPTER 9

Alternatives to Drugs

Psychiatric practice need not depend exclusively on a single tool. For many clinical problems, drugs are not the only (or even the best) form of treatment.

Some alternatives involve other methods of biological treatment. Thus, ECT is an evidence-based alternative for severe depression that is not sufficiently utilized. Other biologically-based options, such as trans-cranial magnetic stimulation and direct brain stimulation, remain experimental.

An alternative suggested by the NICE guidelines for depression is exercise. But depressed patients, who often complain of fatigue, might not follow that recommendation.

9.1 THE EFFICACY AND EFFECTIVENESS OF PSYCHOTHERAPY

The most important (and most under-utilized) alternative to drugs is *psychotherapy*. Psychological treatments have gone into decline in psychiatry, partly because of disillusionment with their effectiveness, and partly because the specialty as a whole has come to see mental illness in the light of neuroscience. (Paris, 2008a). Some psychotherapies tend to go on for years without any proven result. Like drug treatment, psychotherapy was over-hyped and over-sold.

Psychiatrists may not be aware that psychotherapy has an enormous research literature demonstrating its efficacy and effectiveness (Lambert, 2003). This form of treatment can be as evidence-based as any drug. Moreover, psychotherapy need not be lengthy – most of this research shows that it works in six months or less. But in many of the conditions we see, methods have to be specifically designed for the symptoms for which it is prescribed. Not any old talking therapy will do.

A large body of evidence has shown that talking therapies can be efficacious and effective for a wide range of psychological symptoms (Lambert, 2003; Butler *et al.*, 2006). Specifically, psychotherapy, when properly conducted, can be just as effective for many depressed patients as antidepressants (Fisher and Greenberg, 1997; Beck, 2008).

Over 20 years ago, a large-scale clinical trial showed that both CBT and interpersonal therapy (IPT) were as effective as drugs in a population with mild to moderate depression (Elkin *et al.*, 1989). Later research reinforced that conclusion (Thase and Jindal, 2003). Support for the efficacy of psychotherapy in mood and anxiety disorders is supported by decades of research on CBT (Beck, 1986, 2008), as well as on interpersonal psychotherapy (Weissman, 2007).

Psychological methods are also important in other diagnoses. In personality disorders, targeted and specific forms of psychotherapy have been shown to be clearly superior to drug treatment (Paris, 2008c). There is even good evidence that psychotherapy can be a useful adjunct to drug therapy in the most severe mental disorders, such as schizophrenia (Turkington, Kingdon, and Weiden, 2006; Tarrier, 2005) and bipolar disorder (Jones, 2004; Scott *et al.*, 2006).

9.2   HOW PSYCHOTHERAPY WORKS

Talking therapy works in two ways: through "common factors" such as empathy and the provision of hope (Frank and Frank, 1991; Wampold, 2001), as well as through specific techniques, such as those developed by CBT (Beck, 2008).

The specific method of psychotherapy provided seems to be less important than whether treatment is planned out and well structured. In the large-scale trial conducted over two decades ago by the NIMH, there was no difference between the two talking therapy conditions, consistent with a large body of comparative trials of psychotherapy showing that most psychological treatments produce equivalent results (Wampold, 2001). Moreover, the fact that many of the milder cases improved with checkups alone supports the wisdom of the NICE guidelines for depression.

By and large, psychotherapy is more appropriate for patients with less severe forms of illness, which generally carry a less severe genetic load and are more related to environmental stressors. In the common mental disorders of mild anxiety and depression (Goldberg and Huxley, 1992), as well as in personality disorders (Paris, 2008c), substance abuse (Dutra et al., 2007), and bulimia nervosa (Shapiro et al., 2007), the evidence for effective drug treatment is quite weak. On the other hand, there is strong evidence that each of the conditions can respond to evidence-based psychotherapies.

Another advantage of psychotherapy is that it can be used to prevent relapse. In a six-year follow-up study (Fava et al., 2004), CBT performed better than medication maintenance in reducing frequency of relapse from depression. Talking therapy may be more expensive in the short run, but it could be cost-effective in the long run.

9.3 COMBINING DRUGS AND PSYCHOTHERAPY

It has long been known that talking therapies can be effectively combined with drug treatment in depression (Klerman et al., 1974). The efficacy of combined treatment in depression was recently confirmed by a large-scale meta-analysis (Cuijpers et al., 2009). A large-scale naturalistic study of adolescent depression (Curry et al., 2006; March and Vitello, 2009) yielded very similar results, and the same findings emerge in the treatment of anxiety disorders (Otto, Smiths, and Reese, 2005).

There have, however, been a few negative findings. As discussed in Chapter 6, in one arm of the STAR*D study (Thase et al., 2007), patients who did not respond to citalopram were asked to consent to random assignment to either cognitive therapy or alternative pharmacologic strategies. Both had comparable outcomes, and although cognitive therapy was better tolerated, pharmacologic augmentation was more rapidly effective. In another recent study (Kocsis et al., 2009), cognitive therapy was not found to be a powerful adjunct to medication.

But the problem with much of this research is that psychological treatments were added as an afterthought, in environments where drug therapy was preferred. That is not a fair test of the efficacy and effectiveness of combination treatment. We need more studies comparing psychotherapy and drugs, randomly assigned separately and together from the very beginning of treatment, along the lines of the reports of Elkin *et al.* (1989) and of Curry *et al.* (2006).

Drawing on a broad literature, Thase and Jindal (2003) concluded that drugs are usually no better than therapy in mild depression, and that when they don't work, patients should be offered a trial of talking therapy. I would go further. Patients should be offered an informed choice from the very first evaluation. Even when drugs are chosen, it may be useful to delay the first prescription until the patient is seen again. It is surprising how often people feel better after a single interview that offers understanding and hope.

9.4   CHOOSING AMONG ALTERNATIVES

While multiple modalities cover more bases, some patients may benefit from medication alone and some from psychotherapy alone. As we have seen it is difficult to predict the response to antidepressants, with severity of symptoms being the best clue. As for psychotherapy, one cannot consider it unless patients are willing to talk. Those who are aware that depressed feelings arise from interpersonal problems are more likely to be interested. Nemeroff *et al.* (2003) found that patients with histories of childhood trauma (which tends to be associated with adult interpersonal difficulties) did better with psychotherapy than with an antidepressant.

Moreover, many patients have complex psychopathology that is not readily accounted for by diagnoses such as mood disorder. Depressed patients with personality disorders respond less well to antidepressants (Newton-Jones *et al.*, 2006), and there is stronger evidence for psychotherapy than for any medication in these conditions (Paris, 2008c). In diagnoses in which talking therapies have a strong evidence base, such as personality disorders, my practice is to start with psychological treatment and only consider drugs when symptoms are not brought under control.

Such observations point to the importance of taking a life history before prescribing antidepressants – a procedure that psychiatrists used to take for granted, but that has fallen by the wayside in our recent enthusiasm for pharmacological solutions.

9.5 WHY PSYCHOTHERAPY IS NOT PRESCRIBED

Given the vast literature supporting its efficacy and effectiveness, evidence-based psychiatric practice should usually include psychotherapy as an option. In light of research, it seems clear that we should be offering depressed patients a choice – of drugs, psychotherapy, or a combination of both. Why does this not happen in practice?

There are several reasons. One has to do with how psychiatrists are trained and how they prefer to practice. These medical specialists, for whom psychotherapy was once a hallmark of their expertise, now rarely offer this form of treatment. In fact, a survey in the USA showed that psychiatrists are unlikely to provide much formal psychological treatment, above and beyond supportive chats (Mojtabai and Olfson, 2008).

Psychiatrists can also earn much more money by prescribing medication than by conducting psychotherapy. That is true in the USA, where payment comes through managed care, as well as in countries like the UK and Canada where governments insure services.

Lack of expertise in psychotherapy among psychiatrists would not be a problem if patients needing psychological treatment were regularly referred to other professionals – much as orthopedists send their patients to physiotherapists. But these referrals do not occur on anything like a routine basis. Psychiatrists are not even always aware that psychotherapy has something important to offer. And if they are, there are problems with access. In the UK, recent efforts to provide access to CBT through the NHS is a hopeful development. But the small number of psychologists still limits availability.

A second reason has to do with patient preferences. Talking therapy as a whole lost respect when psychoanalysis became discredited by lack of proof for its efficacy (Paris, 2005). CBT and other evidence-based methods have filled the niche, and briefer methods of psychotherapy are more available than in the past (Kessler et al., 2005b). Yet my experience in consultations is that many (if not most) patients with common mental disorders expect drug treatment.

9.6 ACCESS AND QUALITY CONTROL

Only some patients have ready access to skilled psychotherapy. They either have to be wealthy, well insured, or lucky.

Unfortunately, talking therapy has been a very contentious and fragmented field. (That was one reason for the decline in its prestige.) In Britain, attempts have been made to bring all therapists under one umbrella, but there was a split between the widely inclusive United Kingdom Council for Psychotherapy (Tantam, 2006), and the psychoanalytically oriented British Council for Psychotherapy (Balfour and Richards, 2007). Membership in either group remains voluntary, and therapists can practice in any way they please without statutory regulation. In the USA, almost anyone can say they are a psychotherapist, and there are hundreds of "schools" of treatment (Lambert, 2003).

The absence of regulation makes it difficult to determine whether psychotherapy is being carried out on the basis of evidence. Moreover, access to well-trained therapists who can provide empirically supported treatment remains spotty. In the UK, the National Health Service supports evidence-based psychotherapy, at least in principle. There are a number of sites where treatment is well funded, and in which researchers have taken advantage of the large samples being treated (Stiles *et al.*, 2007).

Following publication of the NICE guidelines for the treatment of depression, the NHS has moved to make high quality psychological services even more widely available. But since demand is greater than supply, there are waiting lists, and it is impossible to guarantee treatment for every patient. Needless to say, there is no access problem for obtaining drug treatment.

In the USA, access to psychological treatment is even more difficult. Managed care means that most patients are insured for, at best, an extended evaluation (i.e., a few weeks of treatment), rather than therapy lasting for several months. In Canada, where I work, access is limited by the fact that government insures the services of physicians, but does not pay for the work of psychologists unless they work on salary within a hospital.

9.7 IDEOLOGY AND PRACTICE

Psychiatrists used to define themselves by their broad and integrative knowledge of the biological, psychological, and social factors in mental illness (Engel, 1980). They prided themselves on their ability to conduct detailed and empathic interviews, and to apply an understanding of mental processes to help patients find solutions to life problems. Only a few considered drugs to be their main or only tool. Interest in the person is what made psychiatry unique within medicine.

Yet this very uniqueness created a problem. Psychiatrists did not get the respect of colleagues who were increasingly conducting high-tech medicine. Many were hurt by these attitudes, and tried as much as possible to practice in the same way as other physicians (Paris, 2008a). They aspired to prescribe drugs, and were encouraged to believe that these options were based on the findings of neuroscience.

Thus, psychiatric practice today more closely resembles other medical specialties. Patients are given prescriptions, with less time spent talking. Expertise in drug treatment has come to be seen as our primary skill. When a patient does not respond to pharmacological therapy, the answer tends to be more drugs, or different drugs.

Ideology lies behind such practices. Modern psychiatry has adopted a biological and reductionistic point of view concerning mental phenomena (Gold, 2009). Complex phenomena such as psychological symptoms are seen as rooted in dysfunctions in neural circuitry and/or neurochemistry. Some leading authorities have argued that mental illness is nothing but a problem in applied neuroscience (Insel and Quirion, 2005).

Research has established that psychiatric drugs have profound effects on neurotransmitters, but that may or may not explain how they work. Once again, there is little or no evidence that mental disorders are associated with chemical imbalances. This idea has been highly seductive, and belief in it dies hard.

Neurochemical theories of mental illness have a grain of truth, but biological dysfunctions do not appear *de novo* – environmental stressors can often trigger symptoms. Again, while all mental activity has a neural substrate, cognition, emotion, and behavioral control are higher-order concepts with emergent properties that can only be, at best, partially explained at a cellular or molecular level (Paris, 2009).

Reductionistic psychiatry tends to see every disorder as potentially amenable to expert psychopharmacology. But to seriously consider alternatives to drug treatment, one needs to understand the value of explaining mental phenomena on a *psychological* level. Psychological constructs provide a different kind of information from analysis at a neuronal level.

A psychological perspective on mental illness is also much more likely to consider environmental influences, particularly personal history and current life situation. There are several ways in which genes and biology influence responses to the environment. Research on gene-environment interactions (Rutter, 2006) has shown that genes shape the environments people choose, as well as the intensity of their reactions to stressors. However, there is also research that shows that changes in brain chemistry, structure, and circuitry can be the *result* of psychosocial influences, rather than their cause. Research in epigenomics (Meaney and Szyf, 2005) shows that environments turn on and turn off gene activity, and that genetic information can actually be modified by life events. Thus, genes and environment can never be considered as separate.

Stress-diathesis models explain psychopathology as an *interaction* between biological vulnerability and environmental stressors (Monroe and Simons, 1991). One may not develop symptoms from an adverse life event unless one carries some kind of vulnerability. Similarly, one may never develop a mental disorder, even in the presence of a diathesis, if life presents few difficult challenges.

While clinicians use pharmacological agents to modify diatheses, they can use psychotherapy to moderate the effects of stressors. It has even been shown that psychological treatments can change brain activity, as assessed by imaging methods (Goldapple *et al.*, 2004).

9.8 BRINGING PSYCHOTHERAPY BACK INTO PSYCHIATRIC PRACTICE

Most psychiatrists know little about the psychotherapy research literature. No industry representatives visit their offices to inform them about the latest findings. And medical specialists rarely attend conferences on the subject.

Yet patients deserve the most efficacious treatment, whether that is a drug, a talking therapy, or both. Psychiatrists need to put aside their ideological biases and do what works.

One of the advantages of combining psychotherapy with drug treatment is that psychiatrists who carry out psychological treatment (or refer patients to someone with the expertise to do so) can find themselves prescribing drugs differently. Knowing that patients are receiving another modality of treatment could make practitioners more cautious, allow them to accept that results take time, and encourage them to avoid rushing into over-prescription and polypharmacy.

The main problem with psychological treatment is that it requires expensive human resources and trained personnel. Drugs are cheaper, at least in the short-run. But considering their limitations, factoring long-run issues such as remission and recovery into treatment choices makes sense.

We should also consider that talking therapy can be cost-effective. This treatment does not have to last for years, and brief treatment has a much stronger evidence base (Lambert 2003; Smith, Glass, and Miller, 1980). There is also evidence that access to psychotherapy leads to reduced overall costs for the health system in the long run, mainly because patients are less likely to present further physical complaints that lead to expensive investigative procedures (Gabbard *et al.*, 1997).

Even if psychiatrists do not have the time or the inclination to provide psychotherapy, they can refer their patients to other professionals (such as psychologists) who can provide these services. The parallel would be how orthopedic surgeons work with physiotherapists to help patients recover from physical injuries.

Finally, practitioners should keep in mind that pharmacological treatment itself is more likely to be successful when patients form a strong alliance with the physician. That requires listening skills and empathy. There is no use being an expert on drugs if you don't know how to convince patients to take them.

CHAPTER 10

Medicalizing Distress

The human condition has always involved a degree of suffering. In the past, religion taught people that life was a vale of tears. But modern society does not accept that idea. We prefer to define any form of severe distress as a disease. This process has been called *medicalization* (Conrad, 2007). In the past, depression or anxiety might have been considered as moral failings. People were told to pull their socks up and get on with it. Today, sympathy for the downtrodden trumps sermonizing.

It has also been suggested that the pharmaceutical industry has been involved in "disease mongering" as a way to increase its profits (Moynihan, Heath, and Henry, 2002). It is true that once one accepts the premise that suffering is a medical problem, unhappy people are more likely to be prescribed drugs.

There are also some practical reasons for the medicalization of psychological suffering. It legitimizes troubled states of mind. It also makes it more likely that government or private insurance will pay for treatment of common mental disorders (Conrad, 2007).

Yet as we have already seen, depression cannot be easily separated from unhappiness. Mulder (2008) has criticized talk about an "epidemic" of depression, a conclusion that is based on the findings of epidemiological studies. He argues that the data is artefactual, since "major depression" is not a category of disease, but a cutoff point on a continuous distribution. Research into the effects of drugs (or psychotherapy) on "depression" must take heterogeneity into account.

The problem is much the same for anxiety disorders. Many people experience anxious symptoms from time to time. A good example is how the concept of post-traumatic stress disorder (PTSD) became mixed up with politics. There can be little doubt that *some* people suffer long-term effects from adverse life events. But most people do not (McNally, 1999). Social concern with the ubiquity of trauma medicalizes the consequences of adversities, with the aim of giving them more attention and priority for scarce resources (Stein *et al.*, 2007).

In the mental health field, the medicalizing of distress has sometimes been called "psychiatrization." That term, first used to describe the experiences of refugees (Jovancevic and Knezevic, 2001; Summerfield, 2001), suggests that the very term "post-traumatic stress disorder" serves more of a social purpose than a definition of disease. (By and large, refugees are too busy surviving to be concerned about any symptoms of PTSD.) Similarly, concern about the suffering of war veterans promoted a culture of care centered around this diagnosis (Young, 1997).

By and large, there is no absolute boundary between distress and disease (Kessler *et al.*, 2003). But establishing a cutoff point is still essential. Otherwise life itself becomes the disorder, for which medicine becomes the cure.

10.1 REASONS FOR MEDICALIZATION

The primary reason for medicalization is legitimacy. People more readily accept being physically ill, but there is a continuing stigma to being mentally ill (Corrigan, 2005). For this reason, those who do not want to be stigmatized by a psychiatric diagnosis may want to normalize their distress. Some may simply say, "I am going through a bad patch." Normalization (the converse of medicalization) is a process that explains the large discrepancy between the high prevalence of mental disorders in the community and the much lower frequency of treatment. But sometimes seeing things as normal is the right answer. Psychiatrists should keep in mind that some of the patients they see will have no diagnosis at all.

Some people want to ensure they are considered to be mentally ill. Doing so can establish eligibility for medical treatment and for financial benefits. The last thing they want to hear is that upset feelings are normal.

Psychiatrists are not trained to see depression and anxiety as a normal part of the human condition. On the contrary, the DSM (as well as the ICD) manuals encourage making diagnoses whenever symptoms are prominent, and use definitions that are very inclusive. And that is why using standard diagnostic criteria in large-scale epidemiological research yields such a high overall prevalence of mental disorder.

In the USA, the National Comorbidity Study, using DSM definitions, found the overall lifetime prevalence for any mental disorder to be 50% (Kessler *et al.*, 2005a). Thus, half the population will at some point meet criteria for a psychiatric diagnosis. This conclusion might be considered to be perfectly reasonable, given that everyone meets lifetime criteria for a *medical* diagnosis. One might even take it as good news that half the population will never have a mental disorder. Alternatively, the 50% estimate could be seen as inflated by the inclusion of sub-clinical and normal states of mind that are not really illnesses.

By and large, psychiatrists have a tendency to medicalize distress. And to some extent everyone does – as witnessed by the way diagnoses such as ADHD or depression are thrown around in common parlance. When I read *Psychiatric News*, a newsletter published by the American Psychiatric Association, I never hear that psychiatrists should stick to what they are uniquely trained for – the management of severe mental illness. Instead, there is a constant drumbeat of claims that milder disorders are frequent and undertreated, requiring many more specialists to be trained and funded.

In countries like the UK or Canada, where governments insure services, there is never any lack of work for psychiatrists to do. They always have too many patients – not too few. Specialists may expend effort to limit the number of referrals, and to get other people to share their heavy case load. But in the USA, where insurance is spotty, psychiatrists can actually be looking for patients. Currently there are 40,000 specialists in psychiatry in the USA, mostly concentrated in large cities (Regier *et al.*, 2003). It is not clear whether this large number has contributed to improving the mental health of the population. About half of these psychiatrists conduct solo practice in an office. Thus they have a motive for marketing their services. Moreover, as family doctors provide most antidepressant prescriptions, and as psychologists conduct most psychotherapy, psychiatrists have moved into doing more consultations. Those who choose to compete with other professionals for the care of common mental disorders have an uncertain niche in the mental health care system.

Another reason for medicalizing distress is that every profession likes to feel appreciated, important, or even indispensable. The idea that half the population is afflicted by mental illness reassures psychiatrists about how much they are needed.

A final factor concerns the clientele that psychiatrists treat. If they were to focus on patients whose problems uniquely require the services of a medical specialist, there would be more than enough practitioners to go around. But psychiatrists who work in offices outside hospitals, and choose to take patients with mild disorders (or with life problems only), need to medicalize distress.

Some have disputed this conclusion. A survey of patients in psychoanalysis in the US, Canada, and Australia, treated by a mixture of psychiatrists and psychologists (Doidge *et al.*, 2002) found that the vast majority had DSM-defined disorders. But this finding says more about the over-inclusiveness of the manual than about whether patients receiving psychoanalysis are medically ill.

10.2   WHAT IS A MENTAL DISORDER?

At what level of severity should we diagnose a mental disorder? There can be no question that patients with schizophrenia, bipolar disorder, or melancholic depression are medically ill. But do patients with milder anxiety, mood disorders, or mild substance abuse fall into the same category?

This is not just a theoretical problem. A formal diagnosis usually leads to the prescription of a course of treatment. And today, that treatment is often a drug. It goes without saying that a broad extension of psychiatric diagnosis has been strongly supported by the pharmaceutical industry. Moreover, the values of modern society, which tend to see people as victims of circumstance or chemistry (rather than as morally responsible) support medicalization.

The problem does not only apply to psychiatry. Medicine has absorbed many conditions that lie outside its traditional concern with morbid pathology (Conrad, 2007). Prominent examples include hormone therapy for menopause, infertility treatment for older women, growth hormone treatment for shortness, and drugs for erectile dysfunction.

Within psychiatry, treatment may be offered for sadness and grief (Horwitz and Wakefield, 2007), for shyness (Wakefield, Horwitz, and Schmitz, 2004), or even for periods of rage – a problem that DSM calls "intermittent explosive disorder" (Kessler *et al.*, 2006).

Sometimes medicalization has advantages. For example, alcoholism, when it was considered a moral failing, could not be effectively treated. In the past, moralizing attitudes supported counterproductive interventions – such as prohibition, or the jailing of those who were publicly intoxicated. Viewing alcoholism in a disease model (long advocated by Alcoholics Anonymous) took away moral judgments and made therapy possible.

But opening the door to medicalization has some major downsides. One is stigmatization. Another is an unnecessary dependency on the health care system. Still another is the support of unnecessary medical treatment.

Once again, the best example is depressed mood. The view of depression as a disease is reasonably appropriate for melancholia. But normal problems, such as sadness after a loss, do not fit the model and do not necessarily respond to medical therapy. In such cases, the environment has to change, and time has to pass for people to feel better.

10.3   IS DIAGNOSIS A GUIDE TO TREATMENT?

One of the thorniest problems in psychiatry is how diagnosis becomes a guide to treatment. The DSM system is widely used, even in the UK (Macaskill and Geddes, 1991). This manual was not designed as a treatment manual, but as a consensus document that would provide a convenient (and hopefully scientific) way of classifying mental illness.

Ideally, it would be useful if we had valid categories of illness to guide treatment. Physicians are familiar with that principle from their medical training. Since the time of William Osler (1898), they have aimed to treat diseases rather than symptoms. For example, we can culture the organism that causes an infection, and choose antibiotic therapy by determining sensitivity. Physicians can also distinguish between different types of hypertension based on etiology, and treat each of them differently.

The idea of making therapy diagnosis-specific became much more influential in the 1960s. In the USA, the Food and Drug Administration (FDA) defined diagnosis-based indications for each drug – and licensed them on that basis. One purpose of that system was to put controls on physician behavior. However, as we have seen, practitioners remained free to go their own way (with off-label prescriptions).

Moreover, diagnosis-specific treatment only made sense when disease entities were valid and well understood. Even in internal medicine, categories of illness are not necessarily specific in etiology and pathogenesis. Many drugs, such as anti-inflammatory agents, still target symptoms rather than diseases.

That is about where we are in psychiatry. While diagnoses allow specialists to communicate with each other, they must be understood as provisional categories. They do not correspond to any known etiological and pathogenetic pathways. The patients who meet criteria for current diagnoses are rather heterogeneous. That is one of the reasons why research on pharmacotherapy often yields inconsistent results. Perhaps future generations will, in the light of greater knowledge, find criteria that truly cut nature at its joints.

To maximize reliability, the DSM system asks clinicians to determine whether a patient meets a defined number of criteria. But that does not ensure validity. We can all agree and still be wrong. Nobody knows if the criteria are written properly, or if they can distinguish one category from another. Finding out would require systematic studies of discriminant validity (which have never been carried out).

Moreover, many DSM categories depend on a "Chinese menu approach," in which diagnosis depends on meeting a given (but arbitrary) number of criteria. Since only a few categories have *required* criteria, without which one cannot make a diagnosis, the DSM system has been plagued by massive overlap. DSM actually *encourages* multiple diagnoses. "Comorbidity," that is, overlap between disorders, is an artifact of the system. It does not mean that two separate diseases exist in the same patient.

DSM manuals define mental disorders entirely on the basis of clinical symptoms and course, rather than on endophenotypes, which are almost completely unknown (Gottesman and Gould, 2003). Ghaemi and McHugh (2007) remark archly that this approach makes the DSM system more like a field guide for birdwatchers than a theoretical text in ornithology.

In the absence of deeper knowledge, the DSM system remains popular, even in countries that never officially adopted it. There is nothing wrong with having a field manual that helps you identify psychiatric syndromes. The problem lies with the *reification* of diagnoses – in other words, seeing them not as convenient tags, but as real entities.

A generation has passed since the current DSM system was introduced, and in the course of time these categories have taken on a reality of their own. One can no longer publish a scientific paper on mental disorders without using the manual. Of course, it is important to ensure that scientific findings can be replicated in other populations. Yet the value of diagnosis is often limited, since patients falling into the same category are often too heterogeneous to predict anything about treatment response. The reason is that DSM categories are syndromes, not diseases.

The DSM-IV manual (American Psychiatric Association, 2000) explicitly eschewed any link between diagnosis and treatment. But that statement never prevented clinicians from considering categories such as major depression as an indication for specific pharmacotherapy. It is not always understood the drugs we use are not like antibiotics. Instead they resemble analgesics, producing similar effects on symptoms in entirely different disease categories.

Psychiatry today suffers an epidemic of diagnoses. Each edition of the DSM manual has become larger. It is not clear if inclusiveness is a sign of increased validity or of hubris. Who benefits from an increased number of diagnoses? That partly depends on how medical services are provided. But most psychiatrists in the UK, Europe, and Canada spend most of their time working in public systems, a pattern that has now come to apply to a majority of practitioners in the USA. Thus the main motive of medicalization is not a need for more business.

Instead, the increased number of available diagnoses for mental disorder legitimizes the tasks that psychiatrists already carry out. And while governments may not look at diagnostic codes very carefully, private insurance companies in the USA do. They will not pay for the treatment of adjustment disorders – or personality disorders.

The DSM manual is written by academics, and although it is meant for clinical use, one of the driving forces behind it is research. A disorder under study has to be in the book if a researcher wants to be funded for a grant. Other beneficiaries of a larger manual include advocacy groups, which aim to gain attention for specific disease categories.

All these factors have led to a proliferation of diagnoses. For example, while few psychiatrists ever diagnose a sleep disorder, a large section on this subject was inserted into DSM-IV to satisfy the subspecialists who run sleep clinics.

Drug companies have been pleased with the increase in psychiatric diagnoses. By and large, an increase in categories means that more people are receiving treatment, so that more patients will be prescribed their products.

Some of these problems may be addressed in the forthcoming DSM-V manual (Kupfer, First, and Regier, 2005). Although details remain to be worked out, disorders will now be classified by a combination of categorical and dimensional methods, leaving room for severity ratings. Moreover, comorbidities will be acknowledged by the use of diagnostic spectra, that is, a description of symptoms that cut across categories. However it is unlikely that the manual will be smaller or contain fewer categories of disorder. It will actually be more complicated. Thus it seems unlikely that DSM-V will be clinician-friendly, or any more useful for treatment planning.

10.4 MEDICALIZATION AND PREVALENCE

Epidemiology has a powerful effect on research and practice, as well as on the public perception of psychiatry. Mental disorders as currently defined have a very high prevalence. As we have seen, half the population meets criteria for one category in the course of a lifetime, and about a third do so in the course of any single year (Kessler *et al.*, 2005a).

Some of the findings for specific diagnoses have been striking. It was not surprising to see a high prevalence for common mental disorders. However some less well-known conditions were found to affect many more people than expected. For example, the NCS-R findings suggested that the prevalence of intermittent explosive disorder (IED) is 2.5% (Kessler *et al.*, 2006). Although I do not know of any psychiatrists (outside of forensic specialists) who make this diagnosis very often, after the paper was published, newspapers reported that 12 million Americans were suffering from uncontrolled episodes of rage. The media had a good story that suggested a terrible epidemic, with irate drivers clogging the nation's already crowded roads. Actually, these numbers reflected how many people are easily angered, not how much they were seriously disabled by rage. (There are days when any of us might wonder if we are about to meet criteria for IED.)

The prevalence of more common diagnoses can also be afflicted by over-inclusive criteria. Thus, major depression has been estimated to afflict at least 10% of the population over a lifetime, and a similar prevalence has been found for alcoholism (Kessler *et al.*, 2005a). Yet these numbers depend on whether one accepts the broad definition of major depressive episode, and what the cut-off point is between alcohol use and abuse.

Based on epidemiological studies, personality disorders are diagnosable in over 10% of the community population, both in the USA (Lenzenweger *et al.*, 2007), as well as in the UK (Coid *et al.*, 2006). Even though this is my own area of research, I consider these numbers to be rather inflated (Paris, 2009b).

Some might say that doubts about high prevalence of disorders only reflect the continued stigma attached to mental illness. Including sub-clinical variants might be justified on the grounds that it resembles what other physicians do when they treat non-disordered patients with high cholesterol or glucose (Kessler *et al.*, 2003).

It must be admitted that medicine has evolved in this direction. We think of viral pneumonia as a more severe version of an upper respiratory infection. In the same way, some forms of mental illness could lie on a continuum with common psychological symptoms. We live our lives in and out of states of illness and health.

But while this point of view is reasonable in theory, it leads to problems in practice. Patients do not necessarily seek medical attention for a common cold. And if they do, they come with an expectation of treatment that itself causes trouble. Good doctors will reassure patients and tell them to get more rest and drink fluids. Unfortunately, that does not always happen. Many patients go home with antibiotics – "just in case." Once physicians make a diagnosis, they may feel obligated to offer treatment.

The same problem arises in psychiatry and primary care, in which medicalization leads to false positive diagnoses of depression (Mitchell, Bae, and Rao, 2009). Patients may come in with transient responses to grief and loss, but can be seen as suffering from a mental disorder. Anyone who has had significant symptoms for more than two weeks will actually meet the criteria for major depression. Although there is no evidence that mild depression routinely requires drugs, they may be offered. Thus, all too often, patients are put on antidepressants they do not need. Then, any remission, spontaneous or otherwise, tends to be attributed to the effects of the prescription. And if the patient does not respond, referral to a specialist, followed by switching and augmentation, may be offered to deal with "treatment resistance." Thus, diagnosis, when reified rather than understood as a broad guideline, drives treatment in a direction it need not take.

10.5   SOCIAL ATTITUDES AND MEDICALIZATION

In the modern world, many people feel *entitled* to be healthy and happy. The last century has brought miraculous technological developments to health care. People live much longer, and expect to recover from even the most serious diseases. It is therefore not surprising that many seek a medical "fix" for almost every symptom. The American physician and bioethicist Carl Elliott (2003) has described a wish to rather be "better than well."

Insomnia, sadness, and reduced sexual desire are no longer considered unfortunate facts of life, but targets for therapy. Using an analogy with plastic surgery, Kramer (1993) introduced the term "cosmetic psychopharmacology." Kramer was referring to an observation that antidepressants (or other drugs) can make people more socially competent. While these effects have not received strong empirical support, their very possibility raises issues in medical ethics and philosophy.

The shift from traditional to modern values has been described as "cultural narcissism," that is, a focus on the self and personal experience as opposed to family and community (Twenge and Campbell, 2009). If we had a more traditional view of the human condition, and did not believe in a universal right to happiness, we might be less surprised when antidepressants do not work.

Reductionism, that is, viewing all mental activity and thought at a neuronal level, underlies the world view of modern psychopharmacology. In contrast, viewing mental disorders at a more psychological level would place the limitations of drugs in context, and open up alternatives for treatment. While psychotherapy has a long history of being offered to the "worried well," we now have the data to show that it also works for patients who have moderate to severe mental disorders. Yet it is not being prescribed for these indications.

10.6 MEDICALIZATION AND SERVICE DELIVERY

The medicalization of distress is an issue for resource allocation. There is a cost-benefit to being aggressive about diagnosis. The screening of populations for depression may even be counterproductive (Thombs *et al.*, 2008, since it does not always identify true cases of illness, but attaches diagnoses to people who do not require treatment (Patten, 2008). Sending people identified as depressed to physicians virtually guarantees they will be offered antidepressants. Prescriptions for these agents have already quadrupled (Olfson and Marcus, 2009). Do we want to offer them to everybody who feels unhappy, no matter what the cause?

The medicalization of distress underlies the over-use of psychiatric drugs. The striking success of drugs for severe mental disorders was a heroic moment in the history of medicine. As a result, we lost sight of their more modest effects on common symptoms, and raised hopes for pharmacological solutions for each and every psychological symptom. This illusion goes hand in hand with the over-inclusiveness of current diagnostic systems.

In this light, the fact that many psychological symptoms are not predictably relieved by pharmacotherapy should not be discouraging. Some things in life are *worth* being upset about.

CHAPTER 11

The Future of Psychopharmacology

11.1 THE BENEFITS AND LIMITS OF DRUGS

The message of this book has been that psychiatrists have some very good drugs, but one can expect bad results when good drugs are over-used, prescribed outside of evidence-based indications, and given to the wrong patients. Thus antipsychotics need not be prescribed for mild depression or anxiety. Mood stabilizers need not be prescribed for moodiness. Antidepressants need not be offered for unhappiness. Stimulants need not be prescribed for inattentiveness.

Another problem lies behind these questionable practices. We do not have the drugs we need for many of the problems we see in practice. We are much in the position of psychiatrists in the past, who prescribed barbiturates for psychosis because phenothiazines had not yet been discovered. We need better and more specific agents for severe mental disorders. Until we have drugs for symptoms that are currently refractory to psychopharmacology, we should be cautious about prescribing currently available agents, which are not necessarily the best option.

11.2 THE CULTURE OF PSYCHOPHARMACOLOGY

Psychopharmacology has become a raison d'être for psychiatric practice. The culture of the specialty has come to perceive its work as grounded in neuroscience and an understanding of brain mechanisms

The Use and Misuse of Psychiatric Drugs: An Evidence-Based Critique by Joel Paris
© 2010 John Wiley & Sons, Ltd

(Insel and Quirion, 2005). Yet, as we have seen, the idea that modern therapy can be firmly based on neuroscience is an illusion. It is, at best, a promise for the distant future. We need to be more humble and acknowledge the enormous gap between brain science and our ability to treat patients.

At this point drug treatment remains a clinical art. We do not really know how the agents we use work in the brain. Many current practices are based on clinical experience, and are either untested, or refractory to an evidence-based perspective. Yet because of the belief that drug therapy is usually scientific, ideas are transmitted incautiously, without waiting for solid evidence.

The "lore" of psychopharmacology consists of practices that are discussed in hallways and conferences, usually without the benefit of data. Much discussion takes place about which drug is "better" – even when data shows that differences are minimal. The psychopharmacology culture also tends to support the most aggressive forms of treatment, which often leads to polypharmacy.

No one has carried out a cross-national study of the practice of psychopharmacology. But there could be cultural factors affecting practice. The NICE guidelines suggest that leading British psychiatrists have a more judicious view of what drugs can and cannot do. Across the pond, American psychiatry seems to reflect that nation's "can do" mentality, which can sometimes lead to a lack of caution and judgment.

11.3 DEVELOPING NEW DRUGS

Psychopharmacology is still at its dawn. Current agents are not consistently effective and have many limitations. We badly need new and better drugs, so that future practice can be more effective and more specific.

Several obstacles stand in the way of this goal. The first is cost. It has been estimated that every new drug requires $800 million in investment from start to finish (DiMasi, Hansen, and Grabowski, 2003). One breakthrough drug can recoup such expenses. But blockbusters are the exception in the business. Thus industry has been understandably reluctant to take on expensive gambles. Drug development is a high-risk operation whose success is far from guaranteed. In the short-run, industry sees more profit to be made by marketing "copy-cat" drugs than by developing a new agent from scratch.

An effective new agent with a novel mechanism would benefit industry, physicians, and patients. But we cannot count on pharmaceutical companies to come up with the new drugs that we need. They prefer to develop variants of current agents, and then market them aggressively.

Industry is also sluggish about investing in agents that will not reach a large market. They see little incentive to develop drugs for serious illnesses that affect only a small percentage of the population. While there are profits to be made on new drugs for schizophrenia, bipolar disorder, and severe depression, it is tempting to invest in agents designed for less severe distress – that could be taken by millions of customers.

Moreover, in spite of recent progress in neuroscience, psychopharmacology remains mostly a matter of trial and error. Developing designer molecules that carry out specific neurochemical tasks or that change brain circuits is many decades away. It is possible that drugs of the future will be based on data from whole genome scans, fM-RIs, or measures of cellular pathways mediated by second and third messengers. Yet at this point such scenarios remain unlikely.

Most agents in current use were discovered by serendipity. That is likely to continue to be the case. And by and large, drug development has remained on a plateau since the glory days of the psychopharmacological revolution. We are using updated versions of agents developed half a century ago (or drugs designed for other purposes that have been applied to other indications).

Moreover, there are many lacunae in drug development. New agents are badly needed to manage symptom domains that are inadequately treated. For example, none of the existing drugs available has been able to relieve the negative symptoms of schizophrenia. We also need agents that can do a better job of managing severe depression. The slow and uncertain action of existing antidepressants points to the need to develop a new generation of fast-acting drugs.

There are also several emerging areas of psychopathology for which we lack effective drugs of any kind. For example, impulsivity, a problem seen in disorders ranging from substance abuse to severe personality disorders, is now being treated with drugs developed for other diagnoses – neuroleptics, mood stabilizers, and antidepressants. All these drugs work by sedating patients. When sedated, one is less likely to act on impulse. But if psychiatrists had more specific agents, they would be in a much better position to provide effective treatment. (One can even imagine that if they had drugs for impulsivity, forensic psychiatrists would be flooded with requests for their services.)

Another example is affective instability (see Chapter 5). Emotional dysregulation, a key feature of personality disorders, is generally associated with impulsive behavioral patterns. This pathological process is not known to respond to current agents (which were developed for another purpose). AI is not a variant of bipolar illness, but a separate problem that could greatly benefit from specific drugs for effective management.

11.4   REASONABLE AND UNREASONABLE CRITIQUES OF PSYCHOPHARMACOLOGY

This book has been intended to be a critique "from the inside." I am a psychiatry professor working in the academic mainstream. I have taken pains not to avoid discrediting the impressive accomplishments of psychopharmacology. All psychological problems have neural correlates. And there can be no doubt that in the most severe disorders, effective treatment absolutely requires biological interventions.

Almost everyone in my profession agrees with these principles. Yet strangely, a stubborn minority continues to oppose them. This is the world of "antipsychiatry" (Crossley, 1998).

Psychiatry must be the only medical specialty whose very legitimacy has been questioned. There is no such thing as "antineurology." Nobody has ever suggested that cardiologists or nephrologists should close up shop and give over healing to non-professionals.

This phenomenon demands an explanation. I suggest that antipsychiatry derives from the stigma attached to being mentally ill. Everyone has a mind, and there is no one who does not feel threatened by a challenge to its integrity. In this way, the fear of having a mental disorder is qualitatively different from the fear of developing a cardiovascular illness or cancer. Mental illness is not just a threat to health, but an attack on one's basic integrity as a person. Some people will always feel threatened that some authority is going to declare them mentally ill and carry them off to a hospital. For this reason, resistance to psychiatry and its drugs may never end.

Moreover, antipsychiatry also arose at a specific moment in history (the 1960s), when authority of all kinds fell under suspicion. The idea that medical specialists could decide who was sane or insane naturally came under challenge.

The "lunatic fringe" of antipsychiatry consists of people who believe that the specialty is a conspiracy against human freedom, and that drugs are only used to silence the powerless. Claiming that mental illness is a myth, that psychopharmacology is little but an assault on the brain, and that patients should be encouraged to refuse such treatments, can only be understood as an extreme response to stigma. Even today, the Church of Scientology attacks psychiatry unrelentingly for prescribing drugs. The word "paranoid" only begins to do justice to such views.

Many of the radical opponents of pharmacotherapy reject the reality of mental illness. The idea of treating seriously ill patients without drugs has been supported by a rather unlikely coalition (Crossley, 1998). The antipsychiatry movement has included left-wing intellectual gurus (Michel Foucault) who were suspicious of authority, radical psychoanalysts (RD Laing) who believed that talking can heal anything, and right-wing libertarians (Thomas Szasz) who defended the rights of individuals at all costs.

Many opponents of psychopharmacology favor psychotherapy, and believe that talking is almost always a better alternative than drugs. That position is, at best, naive. Since the seminal work of May (1968), a vast body of evidence has shown that talking (by itself) is almost completely useless for the acute management of psychosis. While there has been some research interest in non-drug treatment for schizophrenia, for example, the "Soteria" therapeutic community program developed by the American psychiatrist Lorne Mosher (Calton *et al.*, 2008), there is little evidence that it works. No one would dream of treating a psychotic patient in that way, even if a few mild cases might get by without maintenance pharmacotherapy. Drug treatment is necessary for almost every patient with an acute psychosis. The role of psychotherapy in the psychoses lies mainly in rehabilitation.

My impression is that antipsychiatrists over-identify with mentally ill patients. Resistance to pharmacology also has a relationship to personal values. Talking to a psychotherapist is more consistent with autonomy and individualism than the more passive experience of taking drugs. Again the key factor is stigma. As long as one is not on medication, one can retain the illusion of being in charge of one's own mind and one's own life.

Confusion has also arisen from the failure to distinguish between the different forms and degrees of mental disorder. For all the problems with psychiatric diagnosis, classification is necessary to plan treatment rationally. Schizophrenia and bipolarity are in a completely different class of illness than common disorders such as anxiety and depression. This book has been mainly critical of prescriptions for people suffering "the sling and arrows of outrageous fortune." Even so, psychotic, manic, and melancholic patients need drugs.

Radical anti-psychiatry is now largely history. The movement's more extreme views have lost favor, and psychiatry has shaken off a concern with politics and social problems. And with time, critics have taken on a more positive role, converting total opposition into the promotion of mental health consumerism (Rissmiller and Rissmiller, 2006).

But with the decline of the prestige of psychotherapy, psychopharmacology emerged as the proverbial last man standing. The social climate underwent a flip-flop in which drugs were valued, while mere talking was looked down on. The educated public came to support pharmacological intervention for psychological symptoms.

By and large, this kind of uninformed and ideologically motivated criticism of psychiatry is a thing of the past. Knowledgeable critics of psychopharmacology have offered much more useful perspectives.

One of the best gadflies is David Healy, a professor at the University of Cardiff and a researcher in the field for decades. While I have disagreements with Healy (discussed in this book), his text "Psychiatric Drugs Explained" (Healy, 2009), is a classic that is now, deservedly, in its fifth edition. This volume stands out for putting modern enthusiasms in context, and demonstrating the limitations of our current armamentarium.

But other critics, while knowledgeable, still manage to be hostile to drugs. Among the most prominent are Joanna Moncrieff, a psychiatrist at University College, London, and her collaborator, Irving Kirsch, a psychologist at the University of Hull. Moncrieff and Kirsch performed a real service by showing that SSRIs are not quite what they are cracked up to be (see Chapter 6). However Kirsch's (2009) view that antidepressants are nothing but placebos (even in severe depression) is an extreme conclusion that offers a serious disservice to depressed patients. A recent book by Moncrieff (2008) is even more "over the top," claiming that antipsychotic drugs are nothing but sedatives that can make the course of psychosis worse, that lithium fails to prevent recurrences of bipolar disorder, and that antidepressants have no role at all in the long-term management of recurrent depression. These critics do not seem to have ever met a drug they don't hate.

The opposition to psychopharmacology is irrational, but it can be partly explained by its strong political flavor. Like the radical psychiatrists of the 1960s, Moncrieff (2008) believes that most patients with mental disorders are suffering from traumatic life events or social oppression. A similar view has come from the British psychologist Richard Bentall, working at Bangor University. In his provocative book entitled *Madness Explained*, Bentall (2003), while not really explaining much about madness, usefully pointed out that drugs do not cure psychosis, that patients who do not like taking these agents are not always wrong, and that psychiatrists are spending very little time with patients obtaining life histories. I can only wish he had stopped there. However Bentall goes on to join the antipsychiatrists, explaining why he distrusts diagnosis, is doubtful of the value of drug treatment, and believes that most psychotic patients are suffering from psychological trauma.

One has to wonder why critics of psychopharmacology can present such uninformed and broadside attacks. Once again, one must invoke the hypothesis that there is something implicitly troubling about medicating the mind.

Yet every field needs gadflies. Psychiatry must come to grips with the challenge of its critics. But I wish these critics would focus less on attacking what we do, and more on the need for better research. For example, Roger Greenberg, a professor of psychology at Syracuse University (Fisher and Greenberg, 1997) who was one of the first to shed doubt on the evidence for antidepressants, emphasized recommendations for different ways of carrying out clinical trials.

11.5   TEACHING PSYCHOPHARMACOLOGY

I have been teaching psychiatry for almost four decades. One of the issues that consistently plagues my students is how to choose the right drug. I have taught them that by and large, they should not worry so much. In almost every case, there are fewer differences between existing agents than they think. But that is not what they hear from their other teachers.

Having lived long enough, I can remember when psychiatrists endlessly discussed the risks and benefits of drugs that are now considered completely equivalent. (Arguments about the efficacy of different tricyclics are now only of historical interest.)

Over several decades, I have been a consultant to family physicians, and I see several hundred cases a year. One of the most frequent questions in these referrals is what to do when patients have failed to respond to an antidepressant (or several antidepressants). The unstated hope is that the right drug or the right group of drugs will do the trick.

While there are times when switching or augmentation should indeed be tried, I am cautious about making such suggestions. As the STAR*D study showed, once two drugs have already been tried, a law of diminishing returns sets in. Moreover, most of the patients sent to me for consultation suffer from poor social supports and lack of success in their work. They have a multitude of real life problems, and many meet criteria for a personality disorder. These clients might benefit more from having access to a psychologist (or a social worker) than from a new prescription.

In presenting these views to students, I find myself working against the grain. Young psychiatrists are not being taught in this way. Their teachers are trapped in a culture that focuses on the hope that even the most refractory patients can be treated with a well-chosen cocktail.

I am worried about where my profession is going, and do not consider that concern to reflect the views of an elderly (and curmudgeonly) professor. There was a time when humanism and understanding were considered essential tools for a psychiatrist. That wasn't enough to help many patients. But psychiatry has gone from one extreme to another.

11.6 WHAT DRUGS CAN AND CANNOT DO

Drugs are essential in psychiatry. They have allowed us to manage severe mental illness and to increase patients' quality of life. It is likely that the drugs of the future will be even more effective.

However, our current armamentarium remains limited, both in scope and in efficacy. We can choose from five major groups: the antipsychotics, the mood stabilizers, the antidepressants, the anxiolytics, and the stimulants. Within these groups, differences between specific agents are relatively minor. And for lack of a better alternative, we are using these drugs for many purposes for which they were not intended, and for which they have not been consistently shown to be effective. We mix and match, fooling ourselves that we are practicing scientific medicine.

This book has taken a hard look at psychopharmacology, and suggested we need to be more humble about what we can and cannot do for patients. No doubt we will be in a position to do more in the future. But for now, we need to set goals that are realistic. Management is not equivalent to cure, but is better than any alternative. Drugs are a powerful tool, but not the only option.

References

Abrams, R. and Taylor, M.A. (1981) Importance of schizophrenic symptoms in the diagnosis of mania. *American Journal of Psychiatry*, **138**, 658–661.

Achenbach, T.M. and McConaughy, S.H. (1997) *Empirically Based Assessment of Child and Adolescent Psychopathology, practical applications*, 2nd edn, Sage Publications, Thousand Oaks, CA.

Ackner, B., Harris, A., and Oldham, A.J. (1957) Insulin treatment in schizophrenia: a controlled trial. *Lancet*, **265**, 607–611.

Akiskal, H.S. (2002) The bipolar spectrum: the shaping of a new paradigm in psychiatry. *Current Psychiatry Reports*, **4**, 1–3.

Akiskal, H.S. (2004) Demystifying borderline personality: critique of the concept and unorthodox reflections on its natural kinship with the bipolar spectrum. *Acta Psychiat Scand*, **110**, 401–407.

Akiskal, H.S. and Benazzi, F. (2003) Family history validation of the bipolar nature of depressive mixed states. *Journal of Affective Disorders*, **73**, 113–118.

Akiskal, H.S. and McKinney, W.T. Jr. (1973) Depressive disorders: toward a unified hypothesis. *Science*, **182**, 20–29.

Akiskal, H.S., Akiskal, K.K., Lancrenon, S. *et al.* (2006) Validating the bipolar spectrum in the French National EPIDEP Study: overview of the phenomenology and relative prevalence of its clinical prototypes. *Journal of Affective Disorders*, **96**, 197–205.

Alda, M. (1999) Pharmacogenetics of lithium response in bipolar disorder. *Journal of Psychiatry and Neuroscience*, **24**, 154–158.

Alda, M. (2009) Is monotherapy as good as polypharmacy in long-term treatment of bipolar disorder? *Canadian Journal of Psychiatry*, **54**, 719–725.

Alphs, R., Anand, R., Islam, M.Z. *et al.* (2004) The International Suicide Prevention Trial (InterSePT): rationale and design of a trial comparing the relative ability of clozapine and olanzapine to reduce suicidal behavior in schizophrenia and schizoaffective patients. *Schizophrenia Bulletin*, **30**, 577–586.

American Psychiatric Association (2000) *Diagnostic and Statistical Manual of Mental Disorders*, 4th edn (text revision), Author, Washington, DC.

American Psychiatric Association (2002) *Practice Guideline for the Treatment of Patients with Major Depressive Disorder*, 2nd edn, American Psychiatric Press, Washington, DC.

American Psychiatric Association (2004) *Practice Guideline for the Treatment of Patients With Schizophrenia*, 2nd edn, American Psychiatric Press, Washington, DC.

Anderson, I.M. (1998) SSRIs versus tricyclic antidepressants in depressed inpatients: A meta-analysis of efficacy and tolerability. *Depression and Anxiety*, **7**(1), 11–17.

Andreasen, N.C. (2001) *Brave New Brain: Conquering Mental Illness in the Era of the Genome*, Oxford University Press, New York.

Andreescu, C., Mulsant, B.H., Peasley-Miklus, C. *et al.* (2007) Persisting low use of antipsychotics in the treatment of major depressive disorder with psychotic features STOP-PD Study Group. *Journal of Clinical Psychiatry*, **68**, 194–200.

Angell, M. (2000) Is academic medicine for sale? *NEJM*, **342**, 1516–1518.

Angell, M. (2005) *The Truth about the Drug Companies: How They Deceive Us and What to Do about It*, Random House, New York.

Angst, J., and Gamma, A. (2002) A new bipolar spectrum concept: a brief review. *Bipolar Disorders*, **4**, 11–14.

Avorn, J. (2004) *Powerful Medicines: The Benefits, Risks, and Costs of Prescription Drugs*, Knopf, New York.

Baastrup, P.C. and Schou, M. (1967) Lithium as a prophylactic agent. Its effect against recurrent depressions and manic-depressive psychosis. *Archives of General Psychiatry*, **16**, 162–172.

Baldessarini, R.J., Ghaemi, S.N., and Viguera, A.C. (2002) Tolerance in antidepressant treatment. *Psychotherapy and Psychosomatics*, **71**, 177–179.

Baldessarini, R.J., Tondo, L., Davis, P. *et al.* (2006) Decreased risk of suicides and attempts during long-term lithium treatment: a meta-analytic review. *Bipolar Disorders*, **8**, 625–639.

Balfour, R. and Richards, J. (2007) History of the British Confederation of Psychotherapists. *British Journal of Psychotherapy*, **11**, 422–426.

Barkley, R. (2006) *Attention-Deficit Hyperactivity Disorder: A Handbook for Diagnosis and Treatment*, 3rd edn, Guilford, New York.

Barratt, A., Wyer, P.C., Hatala, R. *et al.* (2004) Tips for learners of evidence-based medicine: 1. Relative risk reduction, absolute risk reduction and number needed to treat. *Canadian Medical. Association Journal*, **171**, 353–358.

Bauer, M., and Dopfmer, S. (1999) Lithium augmentation in treatment-resistant depression: meta-analysis of placebo controlled studies. *Journal of Clinical Psychopharmacology*, **19**, 427–434.

Bauer, M., Pretorius, H.W., Constant, E.L. *et al.* (2009) Extended-release quetiapine as adjunct to an antidepressant in patients with major depressive disorder: results of a randomized, placebo-controlled, double-blind study. *Journal of Clinical Psychiatry*, **70**, 540–549.

Beck, A.T. (1986) *Cognitive Therapy and the Emotional Disorders*, Basic, New York.

Beck, A.T. (2008) The evolution of the cognitive model of depression and its neurobiological correlates. *American Journal of Psychiatry*, **165**, 969–977.

Beck, S., and Olek, A. (2003) *The Epigenome: Molecular Hide and Seek*, John Wiley & Sons, Ltd, London.

Benedetti, F. (2008) *Placebo Effects: Understanding the Mechanisms in Health and Disease*, Oxford University Press, New York.

Bentall, R.P. (2003) *Madness Explained. Psychosis and Human Nature*, Penguin, London.

Benazzi, F. (2004) Factor structure of recalled DSM-IV hypomanic symptoms of bipolar II disorder. *Comprehensive Psychiatry*, **45**, 441–446.

Berman, R.M., Marcus, R.N., and Swanink, R. (2007) The efficacy and safety of aripiprazole as adjunctive therapy in major depressive disorder: a multicenter, randomized, double-blind, placebo-controlled study. *Journal of Clinical Psychiatry*, **68**, 843–853.

Bhatia, S.K., Rezac, A.J., Vitiello, B. *et al.* (2008) Antidepressant prescribing practices for the treatment of children and adolescents. *Journal of Child and Adolescent Psychopharmacology*, **18**, 70–80.

Binks, C.A., Fenton, M., McCarthy, L. *et al.* (2006) Pharmacological interventions for people with borderline personality disorder. *Cochrane Database of Systematic Reviews* **1** (Art. No.: CD005653). DOI: 10.1002/14651858.CD005653

Birmaher, B., Axelson, D., Goldstein, B., and Strober, M. (2009) Four-year longitudinal course of children and adolescents with bipolar spectrum disorders: The Course and Outcome of Bipolar Youth (COBY) Study. *American Journal of Psychiatry*, **166**, 795–804.

Blier, P. (2008) Do antidepressants really work?. *Journal of Psychiatry & Neuroscience*, **33**, 89–90.

Blier, P., Ward, H.E., Tremblay, P. *et al.* (2010) Combination of antidepressant medications from treatment initiation for major depressive disorder: a double-blind randomized study. *American Journal of Psychiatry*, **167**, 281–288.

Bond, A. (2005) Antidepressant treatments and human aggression. *European Journal of Pharmacology*, **526**, 218–225.

Bowden, C.L. (2007) Spectrum of effectiveness of valproate in neuropsychiatry. *Expert Review of Neurotherapeutics*, **7**, 9–16.

Bowden, C.L., Brugger, A.M., Swann, A.C. *et al.* (1994) Efficacy of divalproex vs lithium and placebo in the treatment of mania. *JAMA*, **271**, 918.

Bowden, C.L., Calabrese, J.R., McElroy, S.L. *et al.* (2000) A randomized, placebo-controlled 12-month trial of divalproex and lithium in treatment of outpatients with Bipolar I disorder. *Archives of General Psychiatry*, **57**, 481–489.

Bowden, C.J., Calabrese, J.R., Sachs, G., Yatham, L.N., Asghar, S.A., Hompland, M., Montgomery, P., Earl, N., Smoot, T.M., DeVeaugh-Geiss, J. for the Lamictal 606 Study Group (2003) A placebo-controlled 18-month trial of lamotrigine and lithium maintenance treatment in recently manic or hypomanic patients with bipolar I disorder. *Arch Gen Psychiatry*, **60**, 392–400.

Braff, D.L., Freedman, R., Schork, N.J., and Gottesman I.I. (2007) Deconstructing schizophrenia: an overview of the use of endophenotypes in order to understand a complex disorder. *Schizophrenia Bulletin*, **33**, 21–32.

Brezo, J., Paris, J., Tremblay, R., Vitaro, F., Hébert, M., Turecki, G. (2007) Distal and proximal correlates of suicide attempts in suicidal ideators: A population-based study. *Psychol Med.*, **37**, 1563–1574.

Brooke, N.S., Wiersgalla, M., and Salzman, C. (2005) Atypical uses of atypical antipsychotics. *Harvard Review of Psychiatry*, **13**, 317–339.

Brotman, M.A., Schmajuk, M., Rich, B.A. *et al.* (2006) Prevalence, clinical correlates, and longitudinal course of severe mood dysregulation in children. *Biological Psychiatry*, **60**, 991–997.

Brunette, M.F., Noordsy, D.L., Xie, H., and Drake, R.E. (2003) Benzodiazepine use and abuse among patients with severe mental illness and co-occurring substance use disorders. *Psychiatric Services*, **54**, 1395–1401.

Butler, A.C., Chapman, J.E., Forman, E.M., and Beck, A.T. (2006) The empirical status of cognitive-behavioral therapy: A review of meta-analyses. *Clinical Psychology Review*, **26**, 17–31.

Cade, J.F.J. (1949) Lithium salts in the treatment of psychotic excitement. *Medical Journal of Australia*, **36**, 349–352.

Calton, T., Ferriter, M., Huband, N., and Spandler, H. (2008) A systematic review of the Soteria paradigm for the treatment of people diagnosed with schizophrenia. *Schizophrenia Bulletin*, **34**, 181–192.

Campbell, E.G., Gruen, R.L., Mountford, J. *et al.* (2007) A national survey of physician–industry relationships. *NEJM*, **356**, 1742–1750.

Carlson, C.L., and Mann, M. (2000) Attention-deficit/hyperactivity disorder, predominantly inattentive subtype. *Child and Adolescent Psychiatric Clinics of North America*, **9**, 499–510.

Caroff, S.N., and Mann, S.C. (1993) Neuroleptic malignant syndrome. *Med Clin North Am*, **77**, 185–202.

Carroll, B.J. (2009) Aripiprazole in refractory depression? *Journal of Clinical Psychopharmacology*, **29**, 90–91.

Carroll, B.J., and Rubin, R.T. (2003) Editorial policies on financial disclosure. *Nature Neuroscience*, **6**, 999–1000.

Casacalenda, N., and Boulenger, J.P. (1998) Pharmacologic treatments effective in both generalized anxiety disorder and major depressive disorder: clinical and theoretical implications. *Canadian Journal of Psychiatry*, **43**, 722–730.

Caspi, A., Moffitt, T.E., Newman, D.L., and Silva, P.A. (1996) Behavioral observations at age three predict adult psychiatric disorders: longitudinal evidence from a birth cohort. *Archives of General Psychiatry*, **53**, 1033–1039.

Caspi, A., McClay, J., Moffitt, T.E. *et al.* (2002) Role of genotype in the cycle of violence in maltreated children. *Science*, **297**, 851–854.

Caspi, A., Sugden, K., Moffitt, T.E. *et al.* (2003) Influence of life stress on depression: moderation by a polymorphism in the 5-HTT gene. *Science*, **301**, 386–389.

Cipriani, A., Barbul, C., and Geddes, J. (2005) Suicide, depression, and antidepressants. *BMJ*, **330**, 373–374.

Cipriani, A., Pretty, H., Hawton, K., and Geddes, J.R. (2005) Lithium in the prevention of suicidal behavior and all-cause mortality in patients with mood disorders: a systematic review of randomized trials. *American Journal of Psychiatry*, **162**, 1805–1819.

Cipriani, A.A., Furukawa, T.A., Salanti, G. *et al.* (2009) Comparative efficacy and acceptability of 12 new-generation antidepressants: a multiple-treatments meta-analysis. *Lancet*, **373**, 746–758.

Cipriani, A., Rendell, J.M., and Geddes, J. (2009) Olanzapine in long-term treatment for bipolar disorder. *Cochrane Database of Systematic Reviews* **21** (**1**) (Art. No.: CD004367). DOI: 10.1002/14651858.CD004367.pub2

Cochrane, A.L. (1972) *Effectiveness and Efficiency. Random Reflections on Health Services*, Nuffield Provincial Hospitals Trust, London.

Collins, A. (1988) *In the Sleep Room*, Lester and Orpen Dennys, Toronto.

Conrad, P. (2007) *The Medicalization of Society*, John Hopkins University Press, Baltimore.

Cooper, J.E., Kendell, R.E., and Gurland, B.J. (1972) *Psychiatric Diagnosis in New York and London*, Oxford University Press, London.

Correll, C.U., Leucht, S., and Kane, J.M. (2004) Lower risk for tardive dyskinesia associated with second-generation antipsychotics: a systematic review of one-year study. *Am J Psychiatry* **161**, 414–425.

Correll, C.U., and Leucht, S. (2007) Weight gain and metabolic effects of mood stabilizers and antipsychotics in pediatric bipolar disorder: a systematic review and pooled analysis of short-term trials. *Journal of the American Academy of Child & Adolescent Psychiatry*, **46**, 687–700.

Corrigan, P.W. (ed.) (2005) *On the Stigma of Mental Illness: Practical Strategies for Research and Social Change*, American Psychological Association, Washington, DC.

Crossley, N.R. (1998) RD Laing and the British anti-psychiatry movement: a socio–historical analysis. *Social Science & Medicine*, **47**, 877–889.

Crystal, S., Olfson, M., Huang, C., Pincus, H., and Gerhard, T. (2009) Broadened use of atypical antipsychotics: safety, effectiveness, and policy challenges. *Health Affairs*, **28**, 770–781.

Cuijpers, P., Dekker, J., Hollon, S.D., and Andersson, G. (2009) Adding psychotherapy to pharmacotherapy in the treatment of depressive disorders in adults: a meta-analysis. *Journal of Clinical Psychiatry*, **70**, 1219–1229.

Cumyn, L., Kolar, D., Keller, A., and Hechtman, L. (2007) Current issues and trends in the diagnosis and treatment of adults with ADHD. *Expert Review of Neurotherapeutics*, **7**, 1375–1379.

Cumyn, L., Hechtman, L., and French, L. (2009) Comorbidity in adults with Attention Deficit Hyperactivity Disorder (ADHD). *Canadian Journal of Psychiatry*, **54**, 673–683.

Curry, J., Rohde, P., Simons, A. *et al.* (2006) Predictors and moderators of acute outcome in the Treatment for Adolescents With Depression Study (TADS). *Journal of the American Academy of Child & Adolescent Psychiatry*, **45**, 1427–1439.

Cutler, A.J., Montgomery, S.A., Feifel, D. *et al.* (2009) Extended release quetiapine fumarate monotherapy in major depressive disorder: a placebo- and duloxetine-controlled study. *Journal of Clinical Psychiatry*, **70**, 526–539.

Dana, J. and Loewenstein, G. (2003) A social science perspective on gifts to physicians from industry. *JAMA*, **290**, 252–255.

Daughton, J.M., Padala, P.R., and Gabel, T.L. (2006) Careful monitoring for agranulocytosis during carbamazepine treatment. *Journal of Clinical Psychiatry: primary care companion*, **8**, 310–311.

DeAngelis, C., Drazen, J.M., Frizelle, F.A. *et al.* (2004) Clinical Trial Registration: A Statement from the International Committee of Medical Journal Editors. *NEJM*, **351**, 1250–1251.

Delay, J., Deniker, P., and Harl, J.-M. (1952) Utilisation en therapeutique psychiatrique d'une phenothiazine d'action. Centrale elective. *Annals of Medicine and Psychology*, **110**, 112–131.

Deshauer, D. (2007) Venlafaxine (Effexor): concerns about increased risk of fatal outcomes in overdose. *CMAJ*, **176**, 39–40.

DeSimoni, M.G., DeLuigi, A., Clavenna, A., and Manfridi, A. (1992) In vivo studies on the enhancement of serotonin reuptake by tianeptine. *Brain Research*, **574**, 93–97.

Deussing, J.M. (2006) Animal models of depression. *Drug Discovery Today: Disease Models*, **3**, 375–383.

DiMasi, J., Hansen, R., and Grabowski, H. (2003) The price of innovation: new estimates of drug development costs. *Journal of Health Economics*, **22**, 151–185.

Doidge, N., Simon, B., Brauer, L. *et al.* (2002) Psychoanalytic patients in the U.S., Canada, and Australia: I. DSM-III-R disorders, indications, previous treatment, medications, and length of treatment. *Journal of the American Psychoanalytic Association*, **50**, 575–614.

Dove, A. (2000) Industry support for medical centers grows. *Nature Medicine*, **6**, 948.

Duffy, A. (2007) Does bipolar disorder exist in children? A selective review. *Canadian Journal of Psychiatry*, **52**, 409–417.

Duffy, A., Alda, M., Hajek, T., and Grof, P. (2009) Early course of bipolar disorder in high-risk offspring: prospective study. *British Journal of Psychiatry*, **195**, 457–458.

Dunbar, G.C., Perere, M.H., and Jenner, F.A. (1989) Patterns of benzodiazepine use in Great Britain as measured by a general population survey. *British Journal of Psychiatry*, **155**, 836–841.

Earle, F. and Mazzacappa, E. (2002) Conduct and oppositional disorders, in *Child and Adolescent Psychiatry* (eds M. Rutter and E. Taylor), John Wiley & Sons, Ltd, London, pp. 419–438.

Eisenberg, L. (2000) Is psychiatry more mindful or brainier than it was a decade ago? *British Journal of Psychiatry*, **176**, 1–5.

Elkin, I., Shea, T., Watkins, J.T., and Imber, S.D. (1989) National Institute of Mental Health Treatment of Depression Collaborative Research Program: general effectiveness of treatments. *Archives of General Psychiatry*, **46**, 971–982.

Elliott, C. (2003) *Better than Well: American Medicine Meets the American Dream*, Norton, New York.

El-Sayeh, H.G.G. and Morganti, C. (2004) Aripiprazole for schizophrenia. *Cochrane Database of Systematic Reviews*, **2** (Art. No.: CD004578), DOI: 10.1002/14651858.

Emanuel, E.J. and Miller, F.G. (2001) The ethics of placebo-controlled trials-a middle ground. *New England Journal of Medicine*, **345**, 915–919.

Engel, G.L. (1980) The clinical application of the biopsychosocial model. *American Journal of Psychiatry*, **137**, 535–544.

Essali, A., Al-Haj Haasan, N., Li, C., Rathbone, J. Clozapine versus typical neuroleptic medication for schizophrenia. Cochrane Database of Systematic Reviews 2009, Issue 1. Art. No.: CD000059. DOI: 10.1002/14651858.CD000059.pub2.

Evidence-Based Medicine Working Group (1992) Evidence-based medicine: a new approach to teaching the practice of medicine. *JAMA*, **268**, 2420–2425.

Faedda, G.L., Baldessarini, R.J., Glovinsky, I.P., and Austin, N.B. (2004) Pediatric bipolar disorder: phenomenology and course of illness. *Bipolar Disorders*, **6**, 305–313.

Faraone, S.V. and Glatt, S.J. (2010) A comparison of the efficacy of medications for adult attention-deficit/hyperactivity disorder using meta-analysis of effect sizes. *Journal of Clinical Psychiatry* Dec 29. [Epub ahead of print], **51**(3), 233–241.

Fava, M. and Davidson, K.G. (1996) Definition and epidemiology of treatment-resistant depression. *Psychiatric Clinics of North America*, **19**, 179–189.

Fava, M. and Rankin, M. (2002) Sexual functioning and SSRIs. *Journal of Clinical Psychiatry*, **63** (suppl 5), 13–16.

Fava, G.A., Ruini, C., Rafanelli, C. *et al.* (2004) Six-year outcome of cognitive behavior therapy for prevention of recurrent depression. *American Journal of Psychiatry*, **161**, 1872–1876.

Fava, G.A. and Rush, J. (2006) Current status of augmentation and combination treatments for major depressive disorder: a literature review and a proposal for a novel approach to improve practice. *Psychotherapy and Psychosomatics*, **75**, 139–153.

Fenton, M., Rathbone, J., Reilly, J., and Sultana, A. (2007) Thioridazine for schizophrenia. *Cochrane Database of Systematic Reviews* **3** (Art. No.: CD001944), DOI: 10.1002/14651858.CD001944.pub2.

Fergusson, D., Doucette, S., and Glass, K.C. (2005) Association between suicide attempts and selective serotonin reuptake inhibitors: systematic review of randomised controlled trials. *BMJ*, **330**, 396–400.

Fink, M. and Taylor, M.A. (2007) Electroconvulsive therapy: Evidence and challenges. *JAMA*, **298**, 330–332.

Fisher, S. and Greenberg, R. (1997) *From Placebo to Panacea: Putting Psychiatric Drugs to the Test*, John Wiley & Sons, Inc., New York.

Flanagin, A. and Rennie, D. (1995) Ghostwriters: not always what they appear. *Journal of the American Medical Association*, **274**, 870–871.

Fournier, J.C., DeRubeis, R.J., Hollon, S.D. *et al.* (2010) Antidepressant drug effects and depression severity: a patient-level meta-analysis. *JAMA*, **303**, 47–53.

Foussias, G. and Remington, R. (2010) Antipsychotics and schizophrenia: From efficacy and effectiveness to clinical decision-making. *Canadian Journal of Psychiatry*, **53**, 117–125.

Frank, J.D. and Frank, J.B. (1991) *Persuasion and Healing*, 3rd edn, Johns Hopkins, Baltimore.

Fraser, L.M., O'Carroll, R.E., and Ebmeier, J.P. (2008) The effect of electroconvulsive therapy on autobiographical memory: A systematic review. *Journal of ECT*, **24**, 10–17.

Freud, S. (1957, Originally published 1896) The aetiology of hysteria, in *The Standard Edition of the Complete Psychological Works of Sigmund Freud*, vol. **3** (ed. and trans. J. Strachey), Hogarth Press, London, pp. 191–224.

Gabbard, G.O., Lazar, S.G., Hornberger, J., and Spiegel, D. (1997) The economic impact of psychotherapy: a review. *American Journal of Psychiatry*, **154**, 147–155.

Gartlehner, G., Gaynes, B.N., Hansen, R.A. *et al.* (2008) Comparative benefits and harms of second-generation antidepressants: Background paper for the American College of Physicians. *Annals of Internal Medicine*, **149**, 734–750.

Gaziano, T.A., Opie, L.H., and Weinstein, M.C. (2006) Cardiovascular disease prevention with a multi-drug regimen in the developing world: a cost-effectiveness analysis. *Lancet*, **368**, 679–686.

Geddes, J.R., Sally Burgess, S., Hawton, K. *et al.* (2004) Long-term lithium therapy for bipolar disorder: systematic review and meta-analysis of randomized controlled trials. *American Journal of Psychiatry*, **161**, 217–222.

Geddes, J.R. for the BALANCE investigators and collaborators (2010) Lithium plus valproate combination therapy versus monotherapy for relapse prevention in bipolar I disorder (BALANCE): a randomised open-label trial. *Lancet*, **375**, 385–395.

Geller, B., Zimerman, B., Williams, M. *et al.* (2002) Phenomenology of prepubertal and early adolescent bipolar disorder: examples of elated mood, grandiose behaviors, decreased need for sleep, racing thoughts and hypersexuality. *Journal of Child & Adolescent Psychopharmacology*, **12**, 3–9.

Geller, B., Tillman, R., Bolhofner, K., and Zimerman, B. (2008) Child bipolar disorder: second and third episodes, predictors of 8-year outcome. *Archives of General Psychiatry*, **65**, 1125–1133.

Ghaemi, S.N. (ed.) (2002) *Polypharmacy in Psychiatry*, Taylor and Francis, Philadelphia.

Ghaemi, S.N., Ko, J.Y., and Goodwin, F.K. (2002) "Cade's disease" and beyond: misdiagnosis, antidepressant use, and a proposed definition for bipolar spectrum disorder. *Canadian Journal of Psychiatry*, **47**, 125–134.

Ghaemi, S.N., Soldani, F. and Hsu, D.J. (2003) Commentary: Evidence-based pharmacotherapy of bipolar disorder. *The International Journal of Neuropsychopharmacology*, **6**, 303–308.

Ghaemi, S.N., and McHugh, P.R. (2007) *The Concepts of Psychiatry*, John Hopkins University Press, Baltimore.

Ghaemi, S.N., Wingo, A.P., Filkowski, M.A., and Baldessarini, R.J. (2008) Long-term antidepressant treatment in bipolar disorder: meta-analyses of benefits and risks. *Acta Psychiatrica Scandinavica*, **118**, 347–356.

Gibbons, R.D., Brown, C.H., and Hur, K. (2007) Early evidence on the effects of regulators' suicidality warnings on SSRI prescriptions and suicide in children and adolescents. *American Journal of Psychiatry*, **164**, 1356–1363.

Gold, I. (2009) Reduction in psychiatry. *Canadian Journal of Psychiatry*, **54**(8), 503–505.

Goldapple, K., Segal, Z., Garson, C. *et al.* (2004) Modulation of cortical-limbic pathways in major depression: treatment-specific effects of cognitive behavior therapy. *Archives of General Psychiatry*, **61**, 34–41.

Goldberg, D. and Huxley, P. (1992) *Common Mental Disorders: A Biopsychosocial Model*, Tavistock Books, London.

Goodwin, F.K., Fireman, B., Simon, G.E. *et al.* (2003) Suicide risk in bipolar disorder during treatment with lithium and divalproex. *JAMA*, **290**, 1467–1473.

Goodwin, F.K. and Jamison, K. (2007) *Manic-Depressive Illness: Bipolar Disorder and Recurrent Depression*, 2nd edn, Oxford University Press, New York.

Gorman, J.M. (1999) Mirtazapine: clinical overview. *Journal of Clinical Psychiatry*, **60**, 9–13.

Gottesman, I. and Gould, T.D. (2003) The endophenotype concept in psychiatry: etymology and strategic intentions. *American Journal of Psychiatry*, **160**, 636–645.

Grad, R. (1997) More evidence linking benzodiazepines and falls. *Canadian Family Physician*, **43**, 1367–1368.

Griesenbach, U., Geddes, D.M. and Alton, E.W. on behalf of the UK Cystic Fibrosis Gene Therapy Consortium (2006) Gene therapy progress and prospects: cystic fibrosis. *Gene Therapy*, **13**, 1061–1067.

Groopman, J. (2007) *How Doctors Think*, Houghton Mifflin, New York.

Gunnell, D., Saperia, J. and Ashby, D. (2005) Selective serotonin reuptake inhibitors (SSRIs) and suicide in adults: meta-analysis of drug company data from placebo controlled, randomised controlled trials submitted to the MHRA's safety review. *BMJ*, **330**, 385–390.

Gupta, S., Mosnik, D., Black, D.W. *et al.* (2004) Tardive Dyskinesia: Review of treatments past, present, and future. *Annals of Clinical Psychiatry*, **11**, 257–266.

Haddad, P. (1998) The SSRI discontinuation syndrome. *Journal of Psychopharmacology*, **12**, 305.

Haddad, P. (1999) Newer antidepressants and the discontinuation syndrome. *Journal of Clinical Psychiatry*, **58**, 17–22.

Hadjipavlou, G., and Yatham, L.N. (2008) Mood stabilizers in the treatment of bipolar II disorder, in *Bipolar II Disorder: Modelling, Measuring and Managing* (ed. G. Parker) Cambridge University Press, Cambridge, pp. 120–137.

Hansen, R., Gaynes, B., Thieda, P. *et al.* (2008) Meta-analysis of major depressive disorder relapse and recurrence with second-generation antidepressants. *Psychiatric Services*, **59**, 1121–1130.

Hatala, R., Keitz, S., Wyer, P., and Guyatt, G. (2005) Tips for learners of evidence-based medicine: 4. Assessing heterogeneity of primary studies in systematic reviews and whether to combine their results. *Canadian Medical Association Journal*, **172**, 661–665.

Hawton, K., Zahl, D. and Weatherall, R. (2003) Suicide following deliberate self-harm: long-term follow-up of patients who presented to a general hospital. *Brit J Psychiatry*, **182**, 537–542.

Healy, D. (1997) *The Antidepressant Era*, Harvard University Press, Cambridge, MA.

Healy, D. (1998) Pioneers in psychopharmacology. *International Journal of Neuropsychopharmacology*, **1**, 191–194.

Healy, D. (2002) *The Creation of Psychopharmacology*, Harvard University Press, Cambridge, MA.

Healy, D. (2004) *Let Them Eat Prozac: The Unhealthy Relationship between the Pharmaceutical Industry and Depression*, New York University Press, New York.

Healy, D. (2008) *Mania: A Short History of Bipolar Disorder*, Johns Hopkins University Press, Baltimore.

Healy, D. (2009) *Psychiatric Drugs Explained*, 5th edn, Elsevier, London.

Healy, D., and Cattell, D. (2003) Interface between authorship, industry and science in the domain of therapeutics. *British Journal of Psychiatry*, **183**, 22–27.

Healy, D., and Thase, M. (2003) Is academic psychiatry for sale? *British Journal of Psychiatry*, **182**, 388–390.

Hechtman, L., Abikoff, H., Klein, R.G. *et al.* (2004) Academic achievement and emotional status of children with ADHD treated with long-term Methylphenidate and multimodal psychosocial treatment. *Journal of the American Academy of Child and Adolescent Psychiatry*, **43**, 812–819.

Heninger, G.R., Delgado, P.L., Charney, D.S., and Hirschfeld, R.M. (1996) The revised monoamine theory of depression. *Pharmacopsychiatry*, **29**, 2–11.

Henry, C., Mitropoulou, V., New, A.S. *et al.* (2001) Affective instability and impulsivity in borderline personality and bipolar II disorders: similarities and differences. *Journal of Psychiatric Research*, **35**, 307–312.

Heres, S., Davis, J., Maino, K. *et al.* (2006) Why olanzapine beats risperidone, risperidone beats quetiapine, and quetiapine beats olanzapine: an exploratory analysis of head-to-head comparison studies of second-generation antipsychotics. *American Journal of Psychiatry*, **163**, 185–194.

Heyman, I., and Fineberg, N.A. (2006) Obsessive-compulsive disorder. *BMJ*, **333**, 424–429.

Hirschfeld, R.M. (1999) Efficacy of SSRIs and newer antidepressants in severe depression: comparison with TCAs. *Journal of Clinical Psychiatry*, **60**, 326–335.

Hodges, B. (1995) Interactions with the pharmaceutical industry: experiences and attitudes of psychiatry residents, interns and clerks. *CMAJ*, **153**, 553–559.

Holbrook, A.M., Crowther, R., Lotter, A. *et al.* (2000) Meta-analysis of benzodiazepine use in the treatment of insomnia. *CMAJ*, **62**.

Horwitz, A.V., and Wakefield, J.C. (2007) *The Loss of Sadness: How Psychiatry Transformed Normal Sorrow into Depressive Disorder*, Oxford University Press, New York.

Inskip, H.M., Harris, E.C., and Barraclough, B. (1998) Lifetime risk of suicide for affective disorder, alcoholism and schizophrenia. *British Journal of Psychiatry*, **172**, 35–37.

Insel, T., and Quirion, R. (2005) Psychiatry as a clinical neuroscience discipline. *JAMA: the journal of the American Medical Association*, **294**, 2221–2224.

Ioannidis, J.P.A. (2005) Why most published research findings are false. *PLoS Med*, **2** (8), e124.

Jayaram, M.B., Hosalli, P., and Stroup, S. (2006) Risperidone versus olanzapine for schizophrenia. *Cochrane Database of Systematic Reviews* **2** (Art. No.: CD005237), DOI: 10.1002/14651858.CD005237.pub2.

Jensen, P.S., Martin, D., and Cantwell, D.P. (1997) Comorbidity in ADHD: Implications for Research, Practice, and DSM-V. *Journal of the American Academy of Child & Adolescent Psychiatry*, **36**, 1065–1079.

Jones, P.B., Barnes, T.R.E., Davies, L. *et al.* (2006) Randomized controlled trial of the effect on quality of life of second- vs first-generation antipsychotic drugs in schizophrenia: Cost Utility of the Latest Antipsychotic Drugs in Schizophrenia Study (CUtLASS 1). *Archives of General Psychiatry*, **63**, 1079–1087.

Jones, S. (2004) Psychotherapy of bipolar disorder: a review. *Journal of Affective Disorders*, **80**, 101–114.

Joy, C.B., Adams, C.E., and Lawrie, S.M. (2006) Haloperidol versus placebo for schizophrenia. *Cochrane Database of Systematic Reviews* **4** (Art. No.: CD003082), DOI: 10.1002/14651858.CD003082.pub2.

Judd, L.L., and Akiskal, H.S. (2003) The prevalence and disability of bipolar spectrum disorders in the US population: re-analysis of the ECA database taking into account subthreshold cases. *Journal of Affective Disorders*, **73**, 123–131.

Judd, L.L., Schettler, P.J., Akiskal, H.S. *et al.* (2008) Residual symptom recovery from major affective episodes in bipolar disorders and rapid episode relapse/recurrence. *Archives of General Psychiatry*, **65**, 386–394.

Juergens, S.M. (1993) Benzodiazepines and addiction. *Psychiatric clinics of North America*, **16** (11), 75–86.

Jureidini, J.N., Doecke, C.J., Mansfield, P.R. *et al.* (2004) Efficacy and safety of antidepressants for children and adolescents. *BMJ*, **328**, 879–883.

Kaymaz, N., VanOs, J., Loonen, A., and Nolen, W.A. (2008) Evidence that patients with single versus recurrent depressive episodes are differentially sensitive to treatment discontinuation: a meta-analysis of placebo-controlled randomized trials. *Journal of Clinical Psychiatry*, **69**, 1423–1436.

Kazdin, A.E. (2005) *Parent Management Training: Treatment for Oppositional, Aggressive, and Antisocial Behavior in Children and Adolescents*, Oxford University Press, New York.

Keck, P.E. Jr., McElroy, S.L., Strakowski, S.M., and Soutullo, C.A. (2000) Antipsychotics in the treatment of mood disorders and risk of tardive dyskinesia. *Journal of Clinical Psychiatry*, **61** (suppl. 4), 33–38.

Kendler, K.S. (2005) Psychiatric genetics: A methodologic critique. *American Journal of Psychiatry*, **162**, 3–11.

Kendler, K.S., and Gardner, C.O. (1998) Boundaries of major depression: An evaluation of DSM-IV criteria. *American Journal of Psychiatry*, **155**, 172–177.

Kendler, K.S., and Prescott, C.A. (2006) *Genes, Environment, and Psychopathology: Understanding the Causes of Psychiatric and Substance Use Disorders*, Guilford Press, New York.

Kerwin, R. (2007) When should clozapine be initiated in schizophrenia? Some arguments for and against earlier use of clozapine. *CNS Drugs*, **21**, 267–278.

Kessler, R.C., Merikangas, K.R., Berglund, P. *et al.* (2003) Mild disorders should not be eliminated from the DSM-V. *Archives of General Psychiatry*, **60**, 1117–1122.

Kessler, R.C., Chiu, W.T., Demler, O. *et al.* (2005a) Prevalence, severity, and comorbidity of 12-month DSM-IV disorders in the National Comorbidity Survey Replication. *Archives of General Psychiatry*, **62**, 617–627.

Kessler, R.C., Coccaro, E.F., Fava, M. *et al.* (2006a) The prevalence and correlates of DSM-IV Intermittent Explosive Disorder in the National Comorbidity Survey Replication. *Archives of General Psychiatry*, **63**, 669–678.

Kessler, R.C., Adler, L., Barkley, R. *et al.* (2006b) The prevalence and correlates of adult ADHD in the United States: Results from the National Comorbidity Survey replication. *American Journal of Psychiatry*, **163**, 716–723.

Ketter, T.A. (2009) Combination therapy versus monotherapy in bipolar disorder. *Journal of Clinical Psychiatry*, **69**, e34.

Khan, A., Khan, S., Kolts, R., and Brown, W.A. (2003) Suicide rates in clinical trials of SSRIs, other antidepressants, and placebo: analysis of FDA reports. *American Journal of Psychiatry*, **160**, 790–792.

Kirsch, I. (2009) *The Emperor's New Drugs: Exploding the Antidepressant Myth*, Random House, London.

Kirsch, I., Deacon, B.J., Huedo-Medina, T.B. *et al.* (2008) Initial severity and antidepressant benefits: a meta-analysis of data submitted to the Food and Drug Administration. *PLoS Med*, **5**, e45.

Klein, D.F. (1978) A proposed definition of mental disorder, in *Critical Issues in Psychiatric Diagnosis* (eds D.F. Klein and R.L. Spitzer), Raven Press, New York, pp. 41–72.

Klein, D.N., and Santiago, N.J. (2003) Dysthymia and chronic depression: introduction, classification, risk factors, and course. *Journal of Clinical Psychology*, **59**, 807–816.

Klerman, G.L. (1990) The psychiatric patient's right to effective treatment: implications of Osheroff v. Chestnut Lodge. *American Journal of Psychiatry*, **147**, 409–418.

Klerman, G.L., DiMascio, A., Weissman, M.M. *et al.* (1974) Treatment of depression by drugs and psychotherapy. *American Journal of Psychiatry*, **131**, 186–191.

Kocsis, J.H. (2003) Pharmacotherapy for chronic depression. *Journal of Clinical Psychology*, **59**, 885–892.

Kocsis, J.H., Gelenberg, A.J., Rothbaum, B.O., and Klein, D.N. (2009) Cognitive behavioral analysis system of psychotherapy and brief supportive psychotherapy for augmentation of antidepressant nonresponse in chronic depression: The REVAMP Trial. *Archives of General Psychiatry*, **66**, 1178–1188.

Koenigsberg, H.W., Harvey, P.D., Mitropoulou, V., Schmeidler, J., New, A.S., Goodman, M., *et al.* (2002) Characterizing affective instability in borderline personality disorder. *American Journal of Psychiatry*, **159**, 784–788.

Koenigsberg, H. (in press) Affective instability: toward an integration of neuroscience and psychological perspectives. *Journal of Personality Disorders.*, **24**(1), 60–82.

Kollins, S.H., Epstein, J.N., and Conners, C.K. (2004) Conners' Rating Scales–Revised, in *The Use of Psychological Testing for Treatment Planning and Outcomes Assessment: Volume 2: Instruments for Children and Adolescents*, 3rd edn (ed. M.E. Maruish), Laurence Erlbaum, Mahwah, NJ, pp. 215–233.

Kollins, S.H., Epstein, J.N., Conners, C.K. (2006) Conners Rating Scale Revised, in M.E. Maruish, *The Use of Psychological Testing for Treatment Planning and Outcomes*, New York, Routledge.

Kowatch, R.A., Fristad, M.A., Birmaher, B. *et al.* (2005) Treatment guidelines for children and adolescents with bipolar disorder. *Journal of the American Academy of Child & Adolescent Psychiatry*, **44**, 213–235.

Kraepelin, E. (1921) *Manic-Depressive Insanity and Paranoia* (Trans. R.M. Barclay, ed. G.M. Robertson), E and S Livingstone, Edinburgh (Original published 1913).

Kramer, P. (1993) *Listening to Prozac*, Viking, New York.

Krueger, R.F. (1999) The structure of common mental disorders. *Archives of General Psychiatry*, **56**, 921–926.

Kuhn, R. (1958) The treatment of depressive states with G 22355 (imipramine hydrochloride). *American Journal of Psychiatry*, **115**, 459–464.

Kupfer, D.J., First, M., and Regier, D. (2005) *A Research Agenda for DSM-V*, American Psychiatric Press, Washington DC.

Kutcher, S.P. (1997) Practitioner review: The pharmacotherapy of adolescent depression, *Journal of Child Psychology and Psychiatry*, **38** (7), 755–767.

Laine, C., Horton, R., DeAngelis, C.D., and Drazen, J.M. (2007) Clinical trial registration: looking back and moving ahead. *CMAJ*, **177**, 1.

Lambert, M. (2003) *Bergin and Garfield's Handbook of Psychotherapy and Behavior Change*, John Wiley & Sons, Inc., New York.

LeCarre, J. (2001) *The Constant Gardener*, Hodder & Stoughton, London.

Lee, P.E., Gill, S.S., Freedman, M. *et al.* (2004) Atypical antipsychotic drugs in the treatment of behavioural and psychological symptoms of dementia: systematic review. *BMJ*, **329**, 75–78.

Lehmann, H.E. (1993) Before they called it psychopharmacology. *Neuropsychopharmacology*, **8**, 291–303.

Lehmann, H.E., and Hanrahan, G.E. (1954) Chlorpromazine, a new inhibiting agent for psychomotor excitement and manic states. *American Medical Association Archives of Neurology and Psychiatry*, **71**, 227–237.

Lenzenweger, M.F., Lane, M.C., Loranger, A.W., and Kessler, R.C. (2007) DSM-IV Personality Disorders in the National Comorbidity Survey Replication. *Biological Psychiatry*, **62**, 553–556.

Leucht, S., Wahlbeck, K., Hamann, J., and Kissling, W. (2003) New generation antipsychotics versus low-potency conventional antipsychotics: a systematic review and meta-analysis. *Lancet*, **361**, 1581–1589.

Leucht, S., Kissling, W., and Davis, J.M. (2009) Second-generation antipsychotics for schizophrenia: can we resolve the conflict? *Psychological Medicine*, **39**, 1603–1606.

Lewis, S., and Lieberman, J.A. (2008) CATIE and CUtLASS: can we handle the truth? *British Journal of Psychiatry*, **192**, 161–163.

Lexchin, J., Bero, L.A., Djulbegovic, B., and Clark, O. (2003) Pharmaceutical industry sponsorship and research outcome and quality: systematic review. *BMJ*, **326**, 1167–1170.

Lexchin, J., and Light, D.W. (2006) Commercial influence and the content of medical journals. *BMJ*, **332**, 1444–1447.

Lieberman, J.A., Stroup, T.S., McEvoy, J.P. *et al.* (2005) Effectiveness of antipsychotic drugs in patients with chronic schizophrenia. *New England Journal of Medicine*, **353**, 1209–1223.

Linehan, M.M. (1993) *Dialectical Behavior Therapy for Borderline Personality Disorder*. New York: Guilford.

Lisman, J.E., Coyle, J.T., Green, R.W. *et al.* (2008) Circuit-based framework for understanding neurotransmitter and risk gene interactions in schizophrenia. *Trends in Neuroscience*, **31**, 234–242.

Lundahl, B., Risser, H.B., and Lovejoy, M.C. (2006) A meta-analysis of parent training: Moderators and follow-up effects. *Clinical Psychology Review*, **26**, 86–104.

Macaskill, N., and Geddes, J. (1991) DSM-III in the training of British psychiatrists: a national survey. *International Journal of Social Psychiatry*, **37**, 182–186.

Macritchie, K., Geddes, J., Scott, J. *et al.* (2001) Valproic acid, valproate and divalproex in the maintenance treatment of bipolar disorder.

Cochrane Database of Systematic Reviews **3** (Art. No.: CD003196), DOI: 10.1002/14651858.CD003196.

MacGillivray, S., Arroll, B., Hatcher, S., and Ogston S. (2003) Efficacy and tolerability of selective serotonin reuptake inhibitors compared with tricyclic antidepressants in depression treated in primary care: systematic review and meta-analysis. *BMJ*, **326**, 1014–1017.

Mannuzza, S., and Klein, R.G. (2000) Long-term prognosis in attention-deficit/hyperactivity disorder. *Child and Adolescent Psychiatric Clinics of North America*, **9**, 711–726.

March, J.S., and Vitello, B. (2009) Clinical messages from the Treatment for Adolescents with Depression Study (TADS). *American Journal of Psychiatry*, **166**, 1118–1123.

Marcus, R.N., McQuade, R.D., and Carson, W.H. (2008) The efficacy and safety of aripiprazole as adjunctive therapy in major depressive disorder. A second, multicenter, randomized, double-blind, placebo-controlled study. *Journal of Clinical Psychopharmacology*, **28**, 156–165.

Maremmani, I., Perugi, G., Pacini, M., and Akiskal, H. (2006) Toward a unitary perspective on the bipolar spectrum and substance abuse: Opiate addiction as a paradigm. *Journal of Affective Disorders*, **93**, 1–12.

Margolese, H., Chouinard, G., Kolivakis, T. *et al.* (2005) Tardive dyskinesia in the era of typical and atypical antipsychotics. Part 1: Pathophysiology and mechanisms of induction. *Canadian Journal of Psychiatry*, **50**, 541–547.

Martinez, C., Rietbrock, S., Wise, L. *et al.* (2005) Antidepressant treatment and the risk of fatal and non-fatal self harm in first episode depression: nested case-control study. *BMJ*, **330**, 389–394.

May, P.R. (1968) *Treatment of Schizophrenia*, Science House, New York.

Mayor, S. (2003) Nature group extends rules on disclosure to review authors. *BMJ*, **327**, 829.

McAlister, F.A. (2008) The "number needed to treat" turns 20 – and continues to be used and misused. *Canadian Medical Association Journal*, **179**, 549–555.

McGee, R.A., Clark, S.E., and Symons, D.K. (2000) Does the Conners' continuous performance test aid in ADHD diagnosis? *Journal of Abnormal Child Psychology*, **28**, 415–424.

McNally, R.J. (1999) Post-traumatic stress disorder, in *Oxford Textbook of Psychopathology* (eds T. Millon, P. Blaney and R. Davis), Oxford University Press, New York, pp. 144–165.

Meaney, M.J., and Szyf, M. (2005) Environmental programming of stress responses through DNA methylation: life at the interface between a dynamic environment and a fixed genome. *Dialogues in Clinical Neuroscience*, **7**, 103–123.

Meltzer, H.Y., Alphs, L., Green, A.I., Altamura, A.C., Anand, R., Bertoldi, A., Bourgeois, M., Chouinard, G., Islam, M.Z., Kane, J., Krishnan, R., Lindenmayer, J.P., Potkin, S. for the InterSePT Study Group (2003) Clozapine treatment for suicidality in schizophrenia International Suicide Prevention Trial (InterSePT) *Arch Gen Psychiatry*, **60**, 82–91.

Merikangas, K.R., Akiskal, H.S., Angst, J. *et al.* (2007) Lifetime and 12-month prevalence of bipolar spectrum disorder in the National Comorbidity Survey replication. *Archives of General Psychiatry*, **64**, 543–552.

Middleton, H., Shaw, I., and Feder, G. (2005) NICE guidelines for the management of depression. *British Medical Journal*, **330**, 267–268.

Miller, E.K., and Cohen, J.D. (2001) An integrative theory of prefrontal cortex function. *Annu Rev Neurosci*, **24**, 167–202.

Miller, W.R., and Carroll, K. (2006) *Rethinking Substance Abuse: What the Science Shows, and What We Should Do about It*, Guilford Press, New York.

Mintzes, B., Morris, L., Barer, R., Kravitz, L., Kazanjian, A., Bassett, K., Lexchin, J., Evans, R.G., Pan, R., Marion, S.R. (2002) Influence of direct to consumer pharmaceutical advertising and patients' requests on prescribing decisions: two site cross sectional survey. *BMJ* **324**, 278–279.

Mitchell, A.J., Bae, A., and Rao, S. (2009) Clinical diagnosis of depression in primary care: a meta-analysis. *Lancet*, **374**, 609–619.

Moeller, F.G., Barratt, E.S., Dougherty, D.M. *et al.* (2001) Psychiatric aspects of impulsivity. *American Journal of Psychiatry*, **158**, 1783–1793.

Mojtabai, R., and Olfson, M. (2010) National trends in psychotropic medication polypharmacy in office-based psychiatry. *Archives of General Psychiatry*, **67**, 26–36.

Moncrieff, J., Wessely, S., Hardy, R. (2004) Active placebos versus antidepressants for depression. *Cochrane Database of Systematic Reviews*, Issue 1. Art. No.: CD003012. DOI: 10.1002/14651858.CD003012.pub2.

Moncrieff, J. (2008) *The Myth of the Chemical Cure*, Palgrave Macmillan.

Moncrieff, J. (2009) A critique of the dopamine hypothesis of schizophrenia and psychosis. *Harvard Review of Psychiatry*, **17**, 214–225.

Moncrieff, J., Wessely, S., and Hardy, R. (2004) Active placebos versus antidepressants for depression. *Cochrane Database of Systematic Reviews* **1** (Art. No.: CD003012), DOI: 10.1002/14651858.CD003012.pub2.

Moncrieff, J., and Kirsch, I. (2005) Efficacy of antidepressants in adults. *BMJ*, **331**, 155–157.

Moncrieff, J., and Cohen, D. (2009) How do psychiatric drugs work? *BMJ*, **338**, 1963.

Monroe, S.M., and Simons, A.D. (1991) Diathesis-stress theories in the context of life stress research. *Psychological Bulletin*, **110**, 406–425.

Montori, V.M., Kleinbart, J., Newman, T.B. *et al.* (2004) Tips for learners of evidence-based medicine: 2. Measures of precision (confidence intervals). *Can. Med. Assoc. J.*, **171**, 611–615.

Moran, M. (2008) Senator wants APA records of drug-industry interactions. *Psychiatric News*, **43** (16), 1.

Moreno, C., Laje, G., Blanco, C. *et al.* (2007) National trends in the outpatient diagnosis and treatment of bipolar disorder in youth. *Archives of General Psychiatry*, **64**, 1032–1039.

Morgan, A.E., Hynd, G.W., Riccio, C.A., and Hall, J. (1996) Validity of DSM-IV ADHD predominantly inattentive and combined types: relationship to previous DSM. *Journal of the American Academy of Child and Adolescent Psychiatry*, **35**, 325–333.

Morgan, J.R. (2002) Review: psychological treatment is as effective as antidepressants for bulimia nervosa, but a combination is best. *Evidence Based Mental Health*, **5**, 75.

Mojtabai, R., and Olfson, M. (2008) National trends in psychotherapy by office-based psychiatrists. *Archives of General Psychiatry*, **65**, 962–970.

Moynihan, R., Heath, I., and Henry, D. (2002) Selling sickness: the pharmaceutical industry and disease mongering. *BMJ*, **324**, 886–891.

Mulder, R.T. (2008) An epidemic of depression or the medicalization of distress? *Perspectives in Biology and Medicine*, **51**, 238–250.

Murphy, B.P., Chung, Y.-C., Park, T.-W., and McGorry, P.D. (2006) Pharmacological treatment of primary negative symptoms in schizophrenia: A systematic review. *Schizophrenia Research*, **88**, 5–25.

National Institute for Health and Clinical Excellence (2006) *The management of bipolar disorder in adults, children and adolescents, in primary and secondary care*. Accessed online, June 2009.

National Institute for Health and Clinical Excellence (2007) *Depression: management of depression in primary and secondary care*. Accessed online, June 2009.

National Institute for Health and Clinical Excellence (2008) *Attention deficit hyperactivity disorder: Diagnosis and management of ADHD in children, young people and adults*. Accessed online, June 2009.

National Institute for Health and Clinical Excellence (2009) *Schizophrenia Core interventions in the treatment and management of schizophrenia in primary and secondary care* (update). Accessed online, May 2009.

Nelson, J.C., Thase, M.E., and Khan, A. (2008) Are antidepressants effective?—what's a clinician to think? *Journal of Clinical Psychiatry*, **69**, 1014–1015.

Nelson, J.C., and Papakostas, G.I. (2009) Atypical antipsychotic augmentation in major depressive disorder: a meta-analysis of placebo-controlled randomized trials. *American Journal of Psychiatry*, **166**, 980–991.

Nemeroff, C.B. (2005) Use of atypical antipsychotics in refractory depression and anxiety. *Journal of Clinical Psychiatry*, **66** (suppl 8), 13–21.

Nemeroff, C.B., and Owens, M.J. (2002) Treatment of mood disorders. *Nature Neuroscience*, **5** (suppl), 1068–1070.

Nemeroff, C.B., and Owens, M.J. (2003) Reply to 'Editorial policies on financial disclosure". *Nature Neuroscience*, **6**, 1000–1001.

Nemeroff, C.B., Heim, C.M., Thase, M.E. *et al.* (2003) Differential responses to psychotherapy versus pharmacotherapy in patients with chronic forms of major depression and childhood trauma. *PNAS*, **100**, 14293–14296.

Nemeroff, C.B., Lieberman, J.A., Weiden, P.J. *et al.* (2005) From clinical research to clinical practice: a 4-year review of ziprasidone. *CNS Spectrums*, **10** (Suppl 17), 1–20.

Nemeroff, C.B., Mayberg, H., Krahl, S.E. *et al.* (2006) VNS therapy in treatment-resistant depression: clinical evidence and putative neurobiological mechanisms. *Neuropsychopharmacology*, **31**, 1345.

Neville, H.J., and Bavelier, D. (2000) Specificity and plasticity in neurocognitive development in humans, in *The New Cognitive Neurosciences*, 2nd edn (ed. M.S. Gazzaniga), The MIT Press, Cambridge, MA, pp. 83–99.

Newcomer, J.W., and Haupt, D.W. (2006) The metabolic effects of antipsychotic medication. *Canadian Journal of Psychiatry*, **51**, 480–491.

Newton-Howes, G., Tyrer, P., and Johnson, T. (2006) Personality disorder and the outcome of depression: meta-analysis of published studies. *British Journal of Psychiatry*, **188**, 13–20.

Norman, T., and McGrath, C. (2000) Stress induced animal models of depression. *Stress Medicine*, **16**, 195–197.

O'Brien, C.P. (2005) Benzodiazepine use, abuse, and dependence. *Journal of Clinical Psychiatry*, **66** (Suppl 2), 28–33.

Ohgami, H., Terao, T., Shiotsuki, I. *et al.* (2009) Lithium levels in drinking water and risk of suicide. *British Journal of Psychiatry*, **194**, 464–465.

Olfson, M., Marcus, S.C., Tedeschi, M., and Wan, G.J. (2006) Continuity of antidepressant treatment for adults with depression in the United States. *American Journal of Psychiatry*, **163**, 101–108.

Olfson, M., and Marcus, S.C. (2009) National patterns in antidepressant medication treatment. *Archives of General Psychiatry*, **66**, 848–856.

Olivieri, N. (2003) Patients' health or company profits? The commercialisation of academic research. *Science and Engineering Ethics*, **9**, 29–41.

Osler, W. (1898) *The Principles and Practice of Medicine*, Applelton, New York.

Otto, M.W., Smiths, J.A.J., and Reese, H.E. (2005) Combined psychotherapy and pharmacotherapy for mood and anxiety disorders in adults: review and analysis. *Clinical Psychology: Science and Practice*, **12**, 72–86.

Owens, E.B., Hinshaw, S.P., and Arnold, L.E. (2003) Which treatment for whom with ADHD? Moderators of treatment response in the MTA. *Journal of Consulting and Clinical Psychology*, **71**, 540–552.

Papakostas, G.I., and Shelton, R.C. (2008) Use of atypical antipsychotics for treatment-resistant major depressive disorder. *Current Psychiatry Reports*, **10**, 481–486.

Parikh, S., LeBlanc, S.R., and Ovanessian, M. (in press) Advancing bipolar disorder: key lessons from the Systematic Treatment Enhancement Program for Bipolar Disorder (STEP-BD). *Canadian Journal of Psychiatry*.

Paris, J. (2005) *The Fall of an Icon: Psychoanalysis and Academic Psychiatry*, University of Toronto Press, Toronto, Ontario, Canada.

Paris, J. (2006) Predicting and Preventing Suicide: Do We Know Enough to Do Either? *Harvard Review of Psychiatry*, **14**, 233–240.

Paris, J. (2008a) *Prescriptions for the Mind*, Oxford University Press, New York.

Paris, J. (2008b) *Treatment of Borderline Personality Disorder: A Guide to Evidence-Based Practice*, Guilford Press, New York.

Paris, J. (2008c) Clinical trials in personality disorders. *Psychiatric Clinics of North America*, **31**, 517–526.

Paris, J. (2009) A critique of the bipolar spectrum. *Harvard Review of Psychiatry*, **17**, 206–213.

Paris, J. (in press) Estimating the prevalence of personality disorders in the community. *Journal of Personality Disorders*.

Paris, J., Gunderson, J.G., and Weinberg, I. (2007) The interface between borderline personality disorder and bipolar spectrum disorder. *Comprehensive Psychiatry*, **48**, 145–154.

Parker, G. (2000) The nature of bipolar depression: implications for the definition of melancholia. *Journal of Affective Disorders*, **59**, 217–224.

Parker, G. (2001) New and old antidepressants: all equal in the eyes of the lore? *British Journal of Psychiatry*, **179**, 95–96.

Parker, G. (2005) Beyond major depression. *Psychological Medicine*, **35**, 467–474.

Parker, G. (ed.) (2008) *Bipolar-II Disorder: Modelling, Measuring and Managing*, Cambridge University Press, Cambridge, UK.

Parker, G. (2009) Antidepressants on trail: how valid is the evidence? *British Journal of Psychiatry*, **193**, 1–3.

Parker, G., Hadzi-Pavlovic, D., and Pedic, F. (1992) Psychotic (delusional) depression: a meta-analysis of physical treatments. *Journal of Affective Disorders*, **24**, 17–24.

Parker, G., and Parker, K. (2003) Which antidepressants flick the switch? A review. *Australian and New Zealand Journal of Psychiatry*, **37**, 464–468.

Parker, G., and Manicavasagar, V. (2005) *Modelling and Managing the Depressive Disorders: A Clinical Guide*, Cambridge University Press, Cambridge, UK.

Patten, S.B. (2008) Major depression prevalence is high, but the syndrome is a poor proxy for community populations' clinical needs. *Canadian Journal of Psychiatry*, **53**, 411–419.

Patten, S.B., and Beck, C.A. (2004) Major Depression and Mental Health Care Utilization in Canada: 1994 to 2000. *Canadian Journal of Psychiatry*, **48**, 303–310.

Patten, S.B., and Paris, J. (2008) The bipolar spectrum—a bridge too far? *Canadian Journal of Psychiatry*, **53**, 762–768.

Pelham, W.E., and Fabian, G.A. (2008) Evidence-based psychosocial treatment for ADHD: An update. *Journal of Clinical Child and Adolescent Psychology*, **37**, 184–214.

Pelkonen, M., and Marttunen, M. (2003) Child and adolescent suicide: epidemiology, risk factors, and approaches to prevention. *Paediatric Drugs*, **5**, 243–265.

Pepper, C.M., Klein, D.N., Anderson, R.L. *et al.* (1995) DSM-III-R Axis II comorbidity in dysthymia and major depression. *American Journal of Psychiatry*, **152**, 239–247.

Perlis, R.H., Perlis, C.S., Wu, Y. *et al.* (2005) Industry sponsorship and financial conflict of interest in the reporting of clinical trials in psychiatry. *Am J Psychiatry*, **162**, 1957–1960.

Perugi, G., and Akiskal, H.S. (2002) The soft bipolar spectrum redefined: focus on the cyclothymic, anxious-sensitive, impulse-dyscontrol, and binge-eating connection in bipolar II and related conditions. *Psychiatric Clinics North America*, **25**, 713–737.

Pini, S., de Queiroz, V., Pagnin, D. *et al.* (2005) Prevalence and burden of bipolar disorders in European countries. *European Neuropsychopharmacology*, **15**, 425–434.

Plomin, R., DeFries, J.C., McClearn, G.E., and Rutter, M.M. (2000) *Behavioral Genetics: A Primer* (3rd ed.). New York: W.H. Freeman.

Preskorn, S.H., and Lacey, R.L. (2007) Polypharmacy: When is it rational? *Journal of Psychiatric Practice*, **13**, 97–105.

Qaseem, A., Snow, V., Denberg, T.D. *et al.* (2008) Using second-generation antidepressants to treat depressive disorders: A clinical practice guideline from the American College of Physicians. *Annals of Internal Medicine*, **149**, 725–733.

Rane, A. (2001) Postgenomic prospects of success in drug development and pharmacotherapy. *Nature, The Pharmacogenomics Journal*, **1**, 6–9.

Ray, W.A., Chung, C.P., Murray, K.T. *et al.* (2009) Atypical antipsychotic drugs and the risk of sudden cardiac death. *NEJM*, **360**, 225–235.

Raz, A. (2006) Perspectives on the efficacy of antidepressants for child and adolescent depression. *PLoS Med*, **3** (1), e9.

Rapoport, J.L., Buchsbaum, M.S., Zahn, T.P. *et al.* (1978) Dextroamphetamine: cognitive and behavioral effects in normal prepubertal boys. *Science*, **199**, 560–563.

Regier, D.A., Wilk, J., West, J.C., and Duffy, F.F. (2003, May) Current status of the psychiatry workforce in the United States. Presented at the American Psychiatric Association, San Francisco.

Rickels, K., Amsterdam, J.D., Clary, C. *et al.* (1991) Buspirone in major depression: a controlled study. *Journal of Clinical Psychiatry*, **52**, 34–38.

Riederer, P., Lachenmayer, L., Laux, G. (2004) Clinical Applications of MAO-Inhibitors, *Current Medicinal Chemistry*, **11**(15), 2033–2044.

Risch, N., Herrell, R., Lehner, T. *et al.* (2009) Interaction between the serotonin transporter gene (5-HTTLPR), stressful life events, and risk of depression: A meta-analysis. *JAMA*, **301**, 2462–2471.

Rissmiller, D., and Rissmiller, J.H. (2006) Evolution of the antipsychiatry movement into mental health consumerism. *Hospital & Community Psychiatry*, **57**, 863–866.

Robins, L. (1966) *Deviant Children Grown Up*. Baltimore, Williams and Wilkins.

Robins, E., and Guze, S.B. (1970) Establishment of diagnostic validity in psychiatric illness: its application to schizophrenia. *American Journal of Psychiatry*, **126**, 107–111.

Rothman, D.J., McDonald, W.J., Berkowitz, C.D. *et al.* (2009) Professional medical associations and their relationships with industry: a proposal for controlling conflict of interest. *JAMA*, **301**, 1367–1372.

Rubinow, D.R. (2006) Depression – augmentation or switch after initial SSRI treatment. *NEJM* **354**, 2611–2613.

Rush, A.J., Fava, M., Wisniewski, S.R. *et al.* (2004) Sequenced Treatment Alternatives to Relieve Depression (STAR*D): rationale and design. *Controlled Clinical Trials*, **25**, 119–142.

Rush, A.J., Trivedi, M.H., Wisniewski, S.R. *et al.* (2006a) STAR*D Study Team: Bupropion-SR, sertraline, or venlafaxine-XR after failure of SSRIs for depression. *New England Journal of Medicine*, **354**, 1231–1242.

Rush, A.J., Wisniewski, S.R., Nierenberg, A.A. *et al.* (2006b) A comparison of mirtazapine and nortriptyline following two consecutive failed medication treatments for depressed outpatients: a STAR∗D report. *American Journal of Psychiatry*, **163**, 1161–1172.

Russell, J., Moskowitz, D., Sookman, D. *et al.* (2007) Affective instability in patients with borderline personality disorder. *J Abnormal Psychology*, **116**, 578–588.

Rutter, M. (2006) *Genes and Behavior: Nature-Nurture Interplay Explained*, Blackwell, London.

Ryan, N.D., Puig-Antich, J., Ambrosini, P. *et al.* (1987) The clinical picture of major depression in children and adolescents. *Archives of General Psychiatry*, **44**, 854–861.

Schachar, R., and Tannock, R. (2002) Syndromes of hyperactivity and attention deficit, in *Child and Adolescent Psychiatry* (eds M. Rutter and E. Taylor), John Wiley & Sons, Ltd, London, pp. 399–418.

Scherk, H., Pajonk, F.G., and Leucht, S. (2007) Second-generation antipsychotic agents in the treatment of acute mania: a systematic review and meta-analysis of randomized controlled trials. *Archives of General Psychiatry*, **64**, 442–455.

Schillevoort, I., de Boer, A., Herings, R.M. *et al.* (2001) Risk of extrapyramidal syndromes with haloperidol, risperidone, or olanzapine. *The Annals of Pharmacotherapy*, **35**, 1517–1522.

Schneider, L.S., Dagerman, K.S., and Insel, P. (2005) Risk of death with atypical antipsychotic drug treatment for dementia: Meta-analysis of randomized placebo-controlled trials. *JAMA*, **294**, 1934–1943.

Schuchman, M. (2005) *The Drug Trial: Nancy Olivieri and the Science Scandal that Rocked the Hospital for Sick Children*, Random House, New York.

Scott, A., Davidson, A., and Palmer, K. (2001) Antidepressant drugs in the treatment of anxiety disorders. *Advances in Psychiatric Treatment*, **7**, 275–282.

Scott, J., Paykel, E., Morriss, R. *et al.* (2006) Cognitive–behavioural therapy for severe and recurrent bipolar disorders: randomised controlled trial. *British Journal of Psychiatry*, **188**, 313–320.

Seeman, P., Lee, T., Chau-Wong, M., and Wong, K. (1976) Antipsychotic drug doses and neuroleptic/dopamine receptors. *Nature*, **261**, 717–719.

Seeman, P., and Kapur, S. (2000) Schizophrenia: More dopamine, more D2 receptors. *PNAS*, **97**, 7673–7675.

Shapiro, J.R., Berkman, N.D., Brownley, K.A. *et al.* (2007) Bulimia nervosa treatment: A systematic review of randomized controlled trials. *International Journal of Eating Disorders*, **40**, 321–336.

Shekelle, P., Maglione, M., Bagley, S. *et al.* (2007) Efficacy and comparative effectiveness of off-label use of atypical antipsychotics. *Comparative Effectiveness Review No. 6.* Rockville, MD: Agency for Healthcare Research and Quality. http://www.rand.org/he (accessed December 2009).

Shelton, C.I. (2004) Long-term management of major depressive disorder: are differences among antidepressant treatments meaningful? *Journal of Clinical Psychiatry*, **65** (Suppl 17), 29–33.

Shepherd, G.M. (1998) *The Synaptic Organization of the Brain*, Oxford University Press, New York.

Shorter, E. (2009) *Before Prozac: the Troubled History of Mood Disorders in Psychiatry*, Oxford University Press, New York.

Shorter, E., and Healy, D. (2007) *Shock Therapy: A History of Electroconvulsive Treatment in Mental Illness*, Rutgers University Press, New Brunswick, N.J.

Singh, M.K., DelBello, M.P., Stanford, K.E. *et al.* (2007) Psychopathology in children of bipolar parents. *Journal of Affective Disorders*, **102**, 131–136.

Sng, J., Meaney, M.J. (2009) Environmental regulation of the neural epigenome. *Epigenomics*, **1**, 131–151.

Srisurapanont, M., Maneeton, B., and Maneeton, N. (2004) Quetiapine for schizophrenia. *Cochrane Database of Systematic Reviews* **2** (Art. No.: CD000967), DOI: 10.1002/14651858.CD000967.pub2.

Stein, D.J., Seedat, S., Iversen, A., and Wessley, S. (2007) Post-traumatic stress disorder: medicine and politics. *Lancet*, **369**, 139–144.

Stiles, W.B., Barkham, M., Twigg, E. *et al.* (2006) Effectiveness of cognitive-behavioural, person-centred and psychodynamic therapies as practised in UK National Health Service settings. *Psychological Medicine*, **36**, 555–566.

Smith, M.L., Glass, G.V., and Miller, T. (1980) *The Benefits of Psychotherapy*, Johns Hopkins Press, Baltimore.

Stafford, R.S. (2008) Regulating off-label drug use—rethinking the role of the FDA. *NEJM*, **358**, 1427–1429.

Stone, M., Laughren, T., Jones, L., Levenson, M., Holland, C., Hugh, A., Hammad, T.A., Temple, R., Rochester, G. (2009) Risk of suicidality in clinical trials of antidepressants in adults: analysis of proprietary data submitted to US Food and Drug Administration. *BMJ*, **339**, b2880.

Summerfelt, W.T., and Meltzer, H.Y. (1998) Efficacy vs. effectiveness in psychiatric research. *Psychiatric Services*, **49**, 834.

Suppes, T., Vieta, E., Liu, S. *et al.* (2009) Investigators maintenance treatment for patients with bipolar I disorder: results from a North American study of quetiapine in combination with lithium or divalproex. *American Journal of Psychiatry*, **166**, 476–488.

Susman, E.J., and Rogol, A. (2004) *Handbook of Adolescent Psychology*, John Wiley & Sons, Ltd, London.

Tamminga, C., and David, J.M. (2007) The neuropharmacology of psychosis. *Schizophrenia Bulletin*, **33**, 937–946.

Tang, T.Z., DeRubeis, R.J., Hollon, S.D. *et al.* (2009) Personality change during depression treatment: A placebo-controlled trial. *Archives of General Psychiatry*, **66**, 1322–1330.

Tantam, D. (2006) Psychotherapy in the UK: Results of a survey of registrants of the United Kingdom Council for Psychotherapy. *European Journal of Psychotherapy, Counselling & Health*, **8**, 321–342.

Tarrier, N. (2005) Cognitive behaviour therapy for schizophrenia – a review of development, evidence and implementation. *Psychotherapy & Psychosomatics*, **74**, 136–144.

Taylor, D. (1989) Current usage of benzodiazepines in Britain. *British Journal of Addiction*, **84**, 541–546.

Thase, M.E. (2008) Do antidepressants really work? A clinicians' guide to evaluating the evidence. *Current Psychiatry Reports*, **10**, 487–494.

Thase, M.E., Entsuah, A.R., and Rudolph, R.L. (2001) Remission rates during treatment with venlafaxine or selective serotonin reuptake inhibitors. *British Journal of Psychiatry*, **178**, 234–241.

Thase, M.E., and Jindal, R.D. (2003) Combining psychotherapy and psychopharmacology for treatment of mental disorders, in *Handbook of Psychotherapy and Behavior Change* (ed. M. Lambert), John Wiley & Sons, Inc., New York, pp. 743–766.

Thase, M.E., Haight, B.R., Richard, N. *et al.* (2005) Remission rates following antidepressant therapy with bupropion or selective serotonin reuptake inhibitors: a meta-analysis of original data from 7 randomized controlled trials. *Journal of Clinical Psychiatry*, **66**, 974–981.

Thase, M.E., Friedman, E.S., Biggs, M.M. *et al.* (2007) Cognitive therapy versus medication in augmentation and switch strategies as second-step treatments: A STAR*D report. *American Journal of Psychiatry*, **164**, 739–752.

The ALLHAT Collaborative Research Group (2002) Major outcomes in high-risk hypertensive patients randomized to angiotensin-converting enzyme inhibitor or calcium channel blocker vs diuretic. *JAMA*, **288**, 2981–2997.

The TADS Team (2007) The Treatment for Adolescents With Depression Study (TADS): Long-term effectiveness and safety outcomes. *Archives of General Psychiatry*, **64**, 1132–1144.

Thieda, P., Beard, S., and Richter, A. (2003) An economic review of compliance with medication therapy in the treatment of schizophrenia. *Psychiatric Services*, **54**, 508–516.

Thombs, B.D., de Jonge, P., Coyne, J.C., and Whooley, M.A. (2008) Depression screening and patient outcomes in cardiovascular care: A systematic review. *JAMA*, **300**, 2161–2171.

Thompson, A., Sullivan, S.A., Barley, M. *et al.* (2008) The DEBIT trial: an intervention to reduce antipsychotic polypharmacy prescribing in adult psychiatry wards – a cluster randomized controlled trial. *Psychological Medicine*, **38**, 705–715.

Tiihonen, J., Lonnqvist, J., Wahlbeck, K. *et al.* (2009) 11-year follow-up of mortality in patients with schizophrenia: a population-based cohort study (FIN11 study). *Lancet*, **364**, 620–627.

Tohen, M., Chengappa, K.N.R., Suppes, T. *et al.* (2006) Relapse prevention in bipolar I disorder: 18-month comparison of olanzapine plus mood stabilizer vs. mood stabilizer alone. *British Journal of Psychiatry*, **184**, 337–345.

Tondo, L., Baldessarini, R., and Floris, G. (2001) Long-term clinical effectiveness of lithium maintenance treatment in types I and II bipolar disorders. *British Journal of Psychiatry*, **178**, s184–s190.

Tone, A. (2008) *The Age of Anxiety*, Basic Books, New York.

Torrens, M., Fonseca, F., Mateu, G., and Farre, M. (2005) Efficacy of antidepressants in substance use disorders with and without comorbid depression. A systematic review and meta-analysis. *Drug & Alcohol Dependence*, **78**, 1–22.

Tost, H., Alam, T., and Meyer-Lindenberg, A. (2009) Dopamine and psychosis: theory, pathomechanisms and intermediate phenotypes. *Neuroscience and Behavioral Reviews* (published on line, June).

Trivedi, M.H., Rush, A.J., Wisniewski, S.R. *et al.* (2006a) Evaluation of outcomes with citalopram for depression using measurement-based care in STAR*D: implications for clinical practice. *American Journal of Psychiatry*, **163**, 28–40.

Trivedi, M.H., Fava, M., Wisniewski, S.R. *et al.* (2006b) Medication augmentation after the failure of SSRIs for depression. *New England Journal of Medicine*, **354**, 1243–1252.

Tsapakis, E.M., Soldani, L., and Baldessarini, R. (2008) Efficacy of antidepressants in juvenile depression: meta-analysis. *British Journal of Psychiatry*, **193**, 10–17.

Turkington, D., Kingdon, D., and Weiden, P.J. (2006) Cognitive behavior therapy for schizophrenia. *American Journal of Psychiatry*, **163**, 365–373.

Turner, E.H., Matthews, A.M., Linardatos, E. *et al.* (2008) Selective publication of antidepressant trials. *NEJM*, **358**, 2180–2182.

Twenge, J.M., and Campbell, W.K. (2009) *The Narcissism Epidemic: Living in the Age of Entitlement*, Simon and Schuster, New York.

Tyrer, P., and Kendall, T. (2009) The spurious advance of antipsychotic drug therapy. *Lancet*, **361**, 1591–1592.

Valenstein, E.S. (1986) *Great and Desperate Cures*, Basic, New York.

Valenstein, E.S. (1998) *Blaming the Brain: The Real Truth About Drugs and Mental Health*, Free Press, New York.

Valenstein, M. (2006) Keeping Our Eyes on STAR*D. *American Journal of Psychiatry*, **193**, 1484–1486.

Valenstein, E.S. (2005) *War of the Soups and the Sparks: The Discovery of Neurotransmitters and the Dispute over How Nerves Communicate*, Columbia University Press, New York.

van Vliet, I.M., den Boer, J.A., and Westenberg, H.W. (1994) Psychopharmacological treatment of social phobia; a double blind placebo controlled study with fluvoxamine. *Psychopharmacology*, **115**, 128–134.

Viguera, A.D., Baldessarini, R.J., and Friedberg, J. (1999) Discontinuing antidepressant treatment in major depression. *Harvard Review of Psychiatry*, **5**, 293–306.

Wakefield, J.C., Horwitz, A.V., and Schmitz, M.F. (2004) Are we overpathologizing the socially anxious? social phobia from a harmful dysfunction perspective. *Canadian Journal of Psychiatry*, **49**, 736–742.

Wakefield, J.C., Schmitz, M.F., First, M.B., and Horwitz, A. (2007) Extending the bereavement exclusion for major depression to other losses. *Archives of General Psychiatry*, **64**, 43–440.

Walsh, B.T., Seidman, S.N., Sysko, R., and Gould, M. (2002) Placebo response in studies of major depression: variable, substantial, and growing. *JAMA*, **287**, 1840–1847.

Wampold, B.E. (2001) *The Great Psychotherapy Debate: Models, Methods, and Findings*, Erlbaum Associates, Mahwah, N.J.

Watanabe, N., Omori, I.M., Nagagawa, A. *et al.* (2008) Mirtazapine versus other antidepressants in the acute-phase treatment of adults with major depression: systematic review and meta-analysis. *Journal of Clinical Psychiatry*, **69**, 1404–1415.

Wazana, A. (2000) Physicians and the Pharmaceutical Industry: Is a gift ever just a gift? *JAMA*, **283**, 373–380.

Weisler, R., Joyce, M., McGill, L. *et al.* (2009) Extended release quetiapine fumarate monotherapy for major depressive disorder: results of a double-blind, randomized, placebo-controlled study. *CNS Spectrums*, **14**, 299–313.

Weiss, G., and Hechtman, L. (1993) *Hyperactive Children Grown Up: ADHD in Children, Adolescents, and Adults*, 2nd edn, Guilford, New York.

Weissman, M.M. (2007) Recent non-medication trials of interpersonal psychotherapy for depression. *The International Journal of Neuropsychopharmacology*, **10**, 117–122.

Westen, D., and Morrison, K. (2001) A multidimensional meta-analysis of treatments for depression, panic, and generalized anxiety disorder: an empirical examination of the status of empirically supported therapies. *Journal of Consulting & Clinical Psychology*, **69**, 875–899.

Whitehead, C., Moss, S., Cardno, A., and Lewis, G. (2003) Antidepressants for the treatment of depression in people with schizophrenia: a systematic review. *Psychological Medicine*, **33**, 589–599. Review: the case for antidepressants for treating depression in people with schizophrenia remains unproven.

Wijkstra, J., Lijmer, J., Balk, F.J., Geddes, J.R., Nolen, W.A. (2006) Pharmacological treatment for unipolar psychotic depression: Systematic review and meta-analysis. *British Journal of Psychiatry*, **188**, 410–5.

Williamson, P. (2006) *Mind, Brain, and Schizophrenia*, Oxford University Press, New York.

Woerner, M.G., Alvir, J.M.J., Saltz, B.L., Lieberman, J.A., and Kane, J.M. (1998) Prospective study of tardive dyskinesia in the elderly: rates and risk factors. *Am J Psychiatry* **155**, 1521–1528.

Woods, J.H., Katz, J.L., and Winger, G. (1988) Use and abuse of benzodiazepines. Issues relevant to prescribing. *JAMA*, **260**, 3476–3480.

World Health Organization (1992) *International Classification of Diseases*, 10th edn, WHO, Geneva.

Wozniak, J. (2005) Recognizing and managing bipolar disorder in children. *Journal of Clinical Psychiatry*, **66** (Suppl 1), 18–23.

Young, A. (1997) *The Harmony of Illusions: Inventing Post-Traumatic Stress Disorder*, Princeton University Press, Princeton, NJ.

Young, S., and Annable, L. (2002) The ethics of placebo in clinical psychopharmacology: the urgent need for consistent regulation. *Journal of Psychiatry & Neuroscience*, **27**, 319–321.

Young, T. (2008) What is the best treatment for bipolar depression? *J Psychiatry Neuroscience*, **33**, 487–488.

Zanarini, M.C., Frankenburg, F.R., Khera, G.S., and Bleichmar, J. (2001) Treatment histories of borderline inpatients. *Comprehensive Psychiatry*, **42**, 144–150.

Zhou, L., Huang, K., Kecojevic, A. *et al.* (2006) Evidence that serotonin reuptake modulators increase the density of serotonin innervation in the forebrain. *Journal of Neurochemistry*, **96**, 396–406.

Zimmerman, M., Ruggero, C.J., Chelminski, I., and Young, D. (2008) Is bipolar disorder overdiagnosed? *Journal of Clinical Psychiatry*, **69**, 935–940.

Zoccolillo, M., Pickles, A., Quinton, D., and Rutter, M. (1992) The outcome of childhood conduct disorder: implications for defining adult personality disorder and conduct disorder. *Psychological Medicine*, **22**, 971–986.

Index

Index compiled by Terry Halliday